Dopamine Detox

Simple Techniques to Take Control Over Your Life

(Simple Techniques to Take Control Over Your Life and Boost Your Focus)

Sharon Swick

Published By **Phil Dawson**

Sharon Swick

Dopamine Detox: Simple Techniques to Take Control Over Your Life (Simple Techniques to Take Control Over Your Life and Boost Your Focus)

ISBN 978-1-998769-58-2

Legal & Disclaimer

Table of contents

Chapter 1: Dopamine Detox (Fast)

A dopamine detox involves replacing low-value activity with high-value activities to create a purposeful, fulfilling existence.

In reality, the term "dopamine detox" is somewhat misleading. Some people call it "dopamine fasting". This is slightly more accurate, but still somewhat off-center.

You can't fasten or detox from dopamine.

Dopamine, which is naturally found in our brains, activates constantly. No matter what you do, dopamine will react to your activity. Simply by reading this, dopamine is being released.

Some words "go untranslatable" when translated into cultural vernacular.

In this example, the words "faster" or "detoxify" mean you are "taking a break" from low-value activities that release powerful neurochemical combinations.

As a result, I'll be using both "fast" (or "detox") interchangeably.

What is dopamine? Is it really important?

Your brain activates neurochemicals to trigger the sequence of events needed for a habit or action.

There are many, however dopamine is our primary focus right now.

Dopamine is a neurotransmitter. This is a chemical within your brain that regulates motivation. It acts as a messenger between your brain cell, sending signals to it whenever it anticipates or is given a "reward."

Dopamine is an important neurochemical. However it is not involved (as many people mistakenly think). It is responsible for motivation, craving, and desiring.

Dopamine plays an important role in the brain's reward mechanism. It helps you recognize things in your environment as vital to your survival. This could relate to:

Feeling good about food, sex, and social status

Dopamine binds directly to "dopamine receivers," which is how dopamine gets into the brain.

Everybody is born with dopaminergic genes. Some people have more dopaminergic receptors than others. Other people have slightly fewer dopaminergic receptors. Most people are somewhere in the middle.

Individuals have unique dopamine receptors that respond to different situations depending on how they are raised, their genes, and the environment in which they live.

Nevertheless, everyone responds to the stimuli almost exactly the same way, with a few exceptions.

Think of it as something as simple as eating some ice cream and playing video games. A majority of people like ice-cream, but many people love playing video games.

However, not everyone loves ice cream. Some prefer video games. Why? Dopamine response can vary depending on other factors.

Although you can become addicted at any time (I had a music obsession), the most common compulsions are those listed above. Every addiction you have is a combination (or variation) of these four.

Dopamine sources can be divided into two types.

Natural Source – Includes eating, drinking, coffee, engaging in sports, and having sex.

Artificial Source – Examples of artificial sources include sugars in junk foods, social networks, or medications.

It is not enough to satisfy, so more is required. Dopamine regulates our daily activities even when it isn't necessary.

What effect does dopamine have upon you?

A positive mood is often associated with a healthy amount of dopamine. It is useful for planning, studying and being productive.

Dopamine creates feelings of:

* Alertness

* Focus

* Motivation

* Happiness

Euphoria can result from a sudden surge in dopamine.

There is both good news and bad news at this moment.

The good news? There aren't many things in the modern world which will instantly kill you.

This is bad news because our brain is not aware of it. Our brains still use evolutionary programming from our ancestors who lived in a rewarding world.

Let's not be naive. Despite our evolution as human beings, we are still very simple creatures. We are fundamentally primordial. You feel amazing when you do something. This is how habits form. Your brain's neuroplasticity can be amazing.

Reinforcement and rewards can train your brain to behave in a particular way. If you have a positive experience, your brain will crave to do it again. Unfortunately, our society of pleasure-addicts can make the hunt for the ultimate dopamine crash a nightmare.

The majority of us live in a rewarding world, especially in the developed nations. This leads to a surprising misalignment of psychology and environment. In this situation, the behavior becomes "overkill", (i.e. The stimuli can lead to addiction.

An addict to food would have survived for 20,000 years. This is because eating too many calories was more preferable than eating too few or enough as there were not many resources. A food addiction can cause death from excessive consumption of sugar, fat and salt, which are all too common.

Even if they didn't pay enough attention, a person addicted to social media would have been able to win because they were constantly looking for new information in the form status updates.

Today, most work is focused. If you lose your focus, it will be difficult to complete tasks. You'll likely be fired soon.

An addict who is able to occasionally reach altered states may have been elevated to the level of a shaman due to their addiction to drugs. They are now just another statistic of the opioid crisis.

All due to dopamine's shift in neurochemical base.

There are several signs that your dopamine levels may be low.

Lack of dopamine may cause you to be unhappy. This could be because you have:

* Low alertness

* Difficulty focusing more on motivation and excitement

* Inadequate coordination may cause mobility difficulties

* Sleep deprivation may reduce dopamine levels.

Dopamine deficiencies can cause sleepiness. However not sleeping can also result in dopamine shortage.

The availability of dopamine receptors during the morning can be affected by sleep deprivation.

Dopamine Fasting & the Neurobiological Baseline

The most important questions that we want to answer during a dopamine detox are:

Is the stimulus something I want to stimulate my brain with dopamine? As mentioned, the purpose of the dopamine fast to stop or eliminate all activities that offer high levels of neurostimulating stimulation at a low cost is to get rid of them.

You will not be more productive if you smoke, use drugs, or consume porn.

These raise your threshold to "acceptable"

You'll feel unfathomable after the first time your use drugs or you have sex. You're on cloud nine. You spend unwittingly days, months and even years trying again to recreate that feeling.

Addiction is the unconscious obsessive reaction to regaining that first high.

Simply put, it is impossible. Why?

Because the brain didn't have anything else to compare the experience with. Your brain is a comparison mechanism that constantly compares this to.

Examples include:

This woman is far more attractive than the other woman.

This food is better than that food.

This vehicle is better than any other vehicle.

In this case, your brain is contrasting low stimulation/high-value activities (work, physical activity, reading, learning, and instrument) with high stimulation/low-value activities (sex, taking drugs, drinking alcohol, watching porn, watching TV, going on social media).

The problem is that activities that generate high value are often boring. They aren't boring but they aren't as stimulating than lower-value activities.

Most likely, you either work or go school. Is it as thrilling as going out for a fun night and getting to know a pretty woman? Most likely not.

To be a valuable employee, you need to have the skills to succeed in your chosen field.

These skills are put into practice and you receive compensation. The reward is only if you work hard (delayedgratification).

But what happens if you get involved in activities that alter your dopaminergic base over time? Activities of low stimulation/high reward become less stimulating.

Activities of low/high value aren't on your radar and you won't be inclined to participate.

High- and low-value activities are incredibly attractive, which makes it more appealing.

Compounded over 5, 10, or even 20 years, this can lead to a life full of lost productivity, addiction, and eventually, a life where you are a slave, rather than a master. You constantly seek pleasure but never receive it. You never seem to find the right thing, even though you're constantly wandering.

To you? You think that is the definition of existence? You're wrong.

The dopamine fast seems like something everyone would do, knowing this.

Even with all of the information, there is still resistance. Even among so-called "educated individuals .".".

Chapter 2: Dopamine Detox Techniques

Dopamine detox is designed for reducing your brain's dependency on non-productive stimuli. There is a way to do it efficiently.

1. Write down all bad habits you have and the origins of them.

A negative habit can be anything that distracts from your goals and hinders your ability to achieve them.

Many people have the major (unconscious!) goal of "living a happy, full and fulfilling life." Although this is a broad goal it's still a worthy one. The majority of your bad habits will affect your enjoyment in the near and long-term.

If financial security is your main prerequisite to a happy lifestyle, then any attempt to undermine that financial stability is a bad idea.

We can go even deeper. Working for a commission can make you money. Being productive at work will help you earn more.

Your work performance can be affected by things like social media use, continuous checking your phone, browsing the Internet, and other activities.

Those are your bad habits.

2. Sort your dopamine-inducing behaviours from most to least important.

These activities consume a lot both time and mental space. These activities are often used for escape.

Drug addicts' subconscious minds are constantly focused on the next time they get high. This means that you are unable to do other things.

But, since most people are not addicted, sex and/or sexual addiction is the next biggest negative behavior. Many men spend their time worrying about the next woman they will have sex with or seeing naked on a monitor. This depletes mental energy that could be used in improving their lives.

This would then be followed by social media, then video games, etc.

3. Take the most difficult choice and give up.

If you're strong enough to do so, you can remove the compulsive one from your life.

If you're able to do it, congratulations. But chances are that you won't succeed because you have forced your brain out homeostasis. It will punish you with horrible cravings and withdrawal and make you feel like it is about time you die.

It is a systematic approach that leads to the most lasting behavioral changes. Progressive approaches focus on staying away of stimuli.

You can't play video games for longer than you have to. This may leave you wondering:

Do you want to slowly wean yourself?

The process of weaning off makes it possible for logic to be used and excuses to be made. You can say:

Just once is enough...

Then, you find yourself back where you started and fighting to stop. You find that your behavior is now more deeply rooted and holds on to you.

Therefore, the best option is to simply give up on it. There will be no more "ifs", or,s. This does not mean that it will ever happen again.

If you drink alcoholic beverages, there's a good chance that you will die. This only applies to behavior addictions. I recommend that you seek professional help if your addiction is severe to alcohol or drugs.

4. You can begin to remove mid-tier pulls.

Next, Things that offer stimulation for prolonged periods of times are decreased. These things are often a drain on mental bandwidth, consuming a lot of time over several weeks, months, or days.

This will be a technology that is accessible to the vast majority of people, which is typical for the attention economy.

These include highly-engaging TV programs, sports season, and even week-long gaming competitions. Watching football can make people spend hours, even days, watching it. These 16 games are part of a regular football season that lasts around 3 hours.

It is easy to get a lot if you multiply that number by the number years or months. Consider gaming contests. You can spend hours playing and preparing for the contests over a period of weeks. It is another waste of time.

Add this to all the other activities in your daily life and it can add up to a lot wasted time on things that really matter.

If you are content in your current position (or retired), this is acceptable. If you're reading these words, you probably want to make progress in your career and achieve your life goals.

You cannot afford to be dragged in for such long periods. You have work to do.

5. Get bored.

When you give up these items, boredom will be your result. Boredom acts as a catalyst to get you moving.

Boredom refers to a sedentary condition. However, humans are constantly looking for ways to move.

The ambient default of a dopamine detox is one of productivity, and honing your personality. As a result you will choose activities that make you a better person now and into the future.

6. Address any emotional issues.

An addiction is a behavior that seeks to fulfill unmet emotional needs. This could include worry, loneliness, or even anger.

You could ask the following questions:

Why did I take this decision?

It is possible that you have been involved in your chosen activity since childhood. Obsessive things are often used as a way to satisfy unmet needs.

Your life is a blurred line if you take drugs, surf the Internet, or watch porn.

Understanding why these behaviors are appealing to you in your daily life is important, regardless of whether they're social anxiety, boredom or lack of friends. You can then create a plan that addresses your emotional gaps, and you will be able to commit to doing what it takes.

7. Begin the process for rewiring and restructuring your brain.

A dopamine detox will help you to organize your brain and reduce dependency on low-value inputs. It will be important to engage and refrain.

You can do this in relative silence (monk-mode), slowly (one out and one in), or all at one time (as previously stated). In any case you'll need a new set of positive behaviors to replace the high/low value behaviors.

It is very unlikely that you will come across anything so intriguing and captivating in the real world.

If you take it out completely, you will create a gap in your psychological life that needs to be filled. While it's possible to eliminate it completely and be "fine", most people don't find it necessary. It is replaced by a system of habits that makes you more productive, engaging and happy.

Dopamine fast requires that you abstain all dopamine-releasing activity. This means you have to do the exact opposite of what you're used to. There is no cellphone. There is not an internet. There aren't clothes. (I promise, the internet is available. If you find a problem behavior, you must eliminate it.

What are you thinking? If it's causing you distress (regarding how much you do), impairment (affects the quality of your social, academic or work performance).

Compulsiveness (a desire to reduce but are unable to consistently do so) There are many ways you can incorporate this practice into daily life. My favorite method is the monthly dopamine rapid.

It's a date on your calendar. Keep track of your days on your wall, even if you don't own a calendar. You will avoid all dopamine on one day each month.

Because the dopamine detox works as a habit-replacement mechanism, it begs the question:

How long does a habit take to develop?

This question is dependent on the difficulty of the habit. A habit of smoking is easier than a habit of meditation.

Smoking is instantaneously addictive and requires little to no thought. Meditation, on the contrary, is more laborious and requires longer observation.

It is possible to meditate for as easy as smoking but this is not realistic in the short-term.

In both cases, you need to be focused on developing positive behaviors that will replace the large number of negative ones and create permanent lifestyle changes.

You must be in it to win it.

Chapter 3: Can A Dopamine Fast Be Used To Quickly Fix Cell Phone Addiction

Many individuals seek out ways to avoid vices that result in poor mental health, such as depression and gorging.

They won't find an all-out deal in dopamine fasting. Berridge discovered that it is a significant part of opposing allurement.

Dopamine fasting, when done properly, is an extraordinary system. He said that "it's just not the absolute arrangement."

Focusing on how to stop enticement has proven to be extremely effective. This can be demonstrated by looking at the treat plate at a gathering and making the decision to leave.

Berridge reminded us that we can't ask the world not to disappear.

The reality is that managing allurements, or pessimistic emotions or behaviors is different from the quick dopamine. Berridge suggested practicing care.

Assisting you in managing the difficult things that you experience each day can be a great way to enjoy every moment of your life.

For practice, the next time that you are feeling tired or going to the internet for entertainment, slow down and notice how your body is responding. Pick another activity to do, all things equal.

What are the Best Things to Do during a Detox?

You are only allowed to read my book. What should you do if fasting is not an option? My days are often filled with walking and light exercise. I also meditate.

The science behind dopamine fasting

Can dopamine "fasting", which is a fasting method, help your mind? Although experts believe so, it's not for the reasons that people may think.

It won't stop the dopamine pathway from being activated for a while (or all) as it does in daily life, but it will be less active.

A misinterpretation about how dopamine works might make it difficult to increase dopamine levels and build joy.

Dopamine had been believed to be the joy chemical many years earlier. It is now understood by specialists how it works, and its subtleties, all the more.

Dopamine is more easily perceived as a substance in our mind that is connected with inspiration. It's vital for us to have a greater prize frame in our cerebrum.

Rewards are things we enjoy and need.

Berridge explained, "The needing and enjoying of these things is independently relegated, dopamine liable for needing."

Consider the case of a notification sound for text messages. It will help you separate this two-layered framework. You can hear the sound going off, but you don't need to know what the text is. It is possible that dopamine has been activated by the warning sound. The message is not likely to bring you joy.

Berridge pointed out that "these [social media] signals" are the perfect little triggers of dopamine frameworks.

Berridge states that dopamine can be used in conjunction with other text to fortify. But it can also cause excessive occupying and upsetting.

He said it is possible to feel attracted to the virtual entertainment that "consistently stimulates a state of need," or one more source of steady dopamine.

What happens to your dopamine levels?

If your dopamine levels are very high, you may feel like you're in the center of the universe for a while.

If it is consumed in excess, it could play a part in:

* mania

* hallucinations

* delusions

Too much dopamine may contribute to:

* Obesity

* Addiction

* Schizophrenia

Low levels of dopamine are associated with the following conditions

Parkinson's disease is characterised by tremors and delayed mobility. In some cases, it can even lead to insanity.

Depression includes sadness, sleep problems, and cognitive abnormalities.

Dopamine transporter deficiency syndrome, commonly known as infantile parkinsonism-dystonia, results in movement disorders akin to Parkinson's disease.

What do drugs have to do with dopamine levels?

Certain medications can interact with dopamine to create a habit. You can activate the dopamine-producing cycle by using substances like nicotine, alcohol or other addictive drugs.

These chemicals can provide dopamine surges that are stronger than those double chocolate chips cookies. You'll want more, and it's so intense that you can't stop wanting more.

When a pattern develops, dopamine levels in the brain decrease. To experience the same pleasure, you now need a large amount of substance.

Over-activation can cause you to lose an interest in other things. This can lead more compulsive behaviour. You lose the ability to stop using these substances.

Addiction happens when you consume more than you need. You might feel physical or mental withdrawal symptoms if you try to stop.

Even if narcotics have been avoided for a while it is possible to get a craving rekindled and even relapse.

Addiction is not caused by dopamine alone. Other factors like genetics and environment also play a significant role in addiction.

Chapter 4: Dopamine Went Wrong

Dopamine does not play a role in this situation. If you didn't have any dopamine, it wouldn't make you feel motivated. They have the potential for being genuine and helpful.

They are evolution's way for you to know that you're doing something good.

Your genes make dopamine the whip that makes you do things. Dopamine highs had been associated with evolutionary benefits until recently. A dopamine rush requires effort and accomplishment.

Instagram was the first time that an elephant was seen to be killed for lunch was the Instagram notification in hunter-gatherer times. Pornography is a woman sleeping in her bed. These two factors increased your chance of survival.

The problem is that dopamine could be used to manipulate it for the wrong reasons. The majority of dopamine hit today offer no real benefit. Instead, these dopamine hits are used to extract more time or money from you. Facebook uses neurochemical strategies to increase your addictive nature. You may be surprised by how often you get notifications. This is to keep your attention occupied and make it more addictive. Brain science also shows that variable reward can increase your addiction potential.

You will still receive random notifications every time Crazy Aunt posts an update to your photo. Dopamine doesn't have a biochemical benefit so you never reach satiation. Here's an example. Hunting for a nice steak would provide dopamine, as well as nutrient sustenance to hunter gatherers. Dopamine levels only increase by visiting the nearest convenience store to indulge in sugary treats. It is easy to get a hit, so you will never feel satisfied. You will find it increasingly difficult to satisfy your cravings the next time. You are now a dopamine addict. This is just like a child with a lighter. It gradually reduces your ability to feel happy and is replaced by a need for meaningful, real-life things. Why be in love with your partner when you could increase engagement through your Instagram profile.

Rewiring Your Brain: Human vs. Monkey

Your brain is being rewired every time you experience a rush of dopamine. Willpower is a muscle even if it is smaller than Charles Barkley's golf game.

Do you hear that voice inside your head telling you not to take drugs? That voice is not common. Two main neural systems are responsible for decision-making: The amygdala controls your monkey brain. (If I had an advanced Harvard degree, I'd refer to this as the A-System). Meanwhile, the prefrontal cortex governs the human mind (sometimes called I System). The Monkey Brain seeks to maximize immediate rewards, while the human one seeks long-term rewards. The monkeys are able to look at the long-term implications of their actions. It is what makes you more successful than just throwing poop at people.

But the monkey brain is still within you. You can't control it. It will rule over you just like Gepetto ruled over Pinocchio.

Think of yourself as staring at a candybar. The internal conflict starts. The internal conflict between your monkey brain and human brains. The monkey inside of you doesn't see the candy. It only thinks about the sweet rush you get from biting into it. "I really do need that candy." "I need it most than anything," you declare to yourself. "That candy bars will change my whole life. "A trained human brain will fight back. Afterward, I'm going be feeling terrible. It's just not worth it. "I must stick to my diet."

You thought the fight of Mike Tyson and Evander Holyfield was big ...?. This is even more. You will lose more than one ear. As any other muscle in the body, the brain too is a muscular. Without proper training, the brain will not fight. Instead of practicing self-control, most people are hitting dopamine buttons. Instead of strengthening willpower, they are making it less strong. It's like going on a gym trip and eating donuts instead of lifting weights.

Too much dopamine makes the balance tip in the monkey's favor. The amygdala becomes hyperactive; the prefrontal cortex becomes passive.

When you do this, you are tightening the strings on your monkey puppetmaster. These systems tend to be short-term-oriented. Your human brain is muted which leads to massive feedback loops. The monkey brain is stronger the more it gets fed.

If you don't have willpower in one part of your life, it is unlikely that you can maintain perfect discipline in the other. How many times have you seen someone meditating and reading a book with a cocaine addiction?

How will you feel after a Dopamine Detox Here are some observations that I have made from dopamine fasts.

My thoughts are still and focused. Your mind is polluted. After dopamine is extracted, it will be like a crystal clear reef.

At times, I crave dopamine. It's almost like my brain is crying out in agony. It actually feels good, oddly. It's a thought that I have been thinking about. It is in my control. It is my responsibility.

I'm experiencing many revelations. Concerning business. Concerning your life. Concerning myself. I believe I have cured cancer, but I forgot to record it. You can remove weeds and allow flowers to blossom.

I am aware of how wasteful these temporary pleasures can be.

More beauty surrounds you. Things that I normally don't notice when I'm on my phone. Even the plants were wonderful. This is why I think vegans should not eat them.

Other Side Effects of Dopamine Addiction

This shift towards the monkey-system has many implications. This doesn't only lead to addictive behaviors but also changes your entire life. A high level of dopamine causes mental obesity. Your brain is no longer able function properly because it has been stuffed full of garbage.

Study: Students have shorter attention spans - The average student has a attention span of 8 seconds, compared to 12 seconds in studies.

Chimpanzees are able to focus on 20 seconds. It's true, humans are much less focused than monkeys. Mind is clutter anxiety. If you don't have enough dopamine, then you get upset.

Do you suffer from constant depression or anxiety? It is possible that your brain has become addicted to dopamine, and your dopamine bar has been reset. You are a heroin addict in your head.

Dominant personality types: Social media excessive use is linked to dysfunctional traits like narcissism and shyness.

Chapter 5: Digital Detox: 6 Tips To Help You Get The Next Digital Cleanse

Technology is everywhere. Americans spend almost half of their time (or 10.5 hours) looking at screens. This is a growing trend in recent years. Although this unprecedented level of information and entertainment access has many benefits, there are also some downsides.

Our social skills, physical and psychological health, and use of social media for entertainment and communication have been harmed. This could also be affecting our children's ability to develop.

Digital detox is a time when we can unplug and disconnect our technology.

Too Much Technology is a Dangerous Trend

While "internet dependency" is not officially recognized by the medical community, there are strong evidence to suggest that excessive screen-time can contribute to poor health, diminished social skills, and the onset or progression of many mental conditions.

Worse, the technology we use seems to have a particular negative effect on our kids. For decades, the long-term implications of being the first generation in our society to have unlimited access and use technology may not be evident.

Too Much Technology: Dangerous Trends

While "internet addict" is not officially recognized by the medical community as a condition, there is ample evidence that excessive screen usage can lead to poor health and impaired social skills. It can also cause mental health problems such as depression, anxiety, and other issues. Worse yet, technology appears to have a particularly harmful impact on our children. For decades, the long-term implications of being the first generation in our society to have unlimited access and use technology may not be evident.

Here are a few examples that technology has an impact on our health and well-being.

Attention is less

Poor memory is caused by a decreased attention span. Social media has made it difficult to pay attention. We're conditioned to expect only short bursts with interesting data and to quickly switch between different sources of data.

People who spend a lot time on the Internet are more likely than others to forget important dates and names. This can have a particularly strong impact on teenagers and children. According to a study, increased digital media use is linked to a rise in symptoms that are comparable to those seen in attention-deficit/hyperactivity disorder (ADHD).

ADHD is a genetic disorder. Too much screen time can make it worse. Your brain reacts to the stimulation and alarm sounds from your device. This can lead you to be obsessive and have high levels of stimulation. Research shows that you're more likely to experience these symptoms if you're younger.

Poor Social Skills

The lack of social skills may also be a negative side effect of media excess exposure. This could be linked to the lack of attention and recall. We are less likely to develop strong social relationships the more we separate from ourselves. Even in crowded public places, our time spent on smartphones, computers, or watching television is not enough to keep us connected.

As we become more familiar with digital interactions, we may lose some of the social skills necessary to communicate in healthy and constructive ways. This can be explained by the loss of physical indicators, such as body language and eye movement. Another reason is people's tendency in the digital age to project often-false personas.

It's been proven that online people can present themselves in a different way than they do in person. Our ability to decide how we want to present ourselves online has led us to have a different view of the world. A digital detox is a way to be present and create meaningful, healthy relationships with others.

Memory Impairment

The amount of information we receive is three times greater than it was 50 years ago. It's becoming harder to differentiate the important from the unimportant with so much information at our disposal. Multitasking has become a norm. Studies show that it reduces our ability for information retention.

Furthermore, most people are able to find the information they require in seconds. We don't need to store as much. Before cell phones we used to remember dozens of numbers. These numbers were for family, friends, colleagues, the doctor, etc. Now that everything is accessible with just a few taps, it's almost impossible to forget them.

It is essential to exercise and cultivate memory. As we age it becomes harder to recover. A digital detox is a great way to improve this skill.

Anxiety, Stress and Depression

Bad social bonding, combined with technological rewiring of the brains has caused a significant increase of stress and anxiety. Many people use their gadgets to deal with stress. Reading emails and playing video games can help release small amounts of dopamine into the brain's pleasure centers.

This can lead to more anxiety, stress, and dependency. We become addicted these short pleasures, seeking more. This damage our dopamine receptors. It perpetuates an endless cycle in which we never have enough.

The compulsive urge to search for missing alerts or new information can cause us to have a constant need to find it. FOMO is a form of anxiety that can be caused by the fear of missing out on important information (FOMO) or a misplaced phone.

Depression

Depression is one side effect of too many technological devices.

Instead of benefitting by real interactions that foster empathy and support each other, we tend to isolate our selves in the warm glow of our screens. The problem is that we only see what is happening in others' lives.

This can make us feel insecure and alone. We start to believe our feelings and emotions may be out of the ordinary, and that no one else feels like we do.

We dig through endless amounts data, exposed to all the extremes of life. The most stunning vacations. The most inspiring stories. The most heartbreaking stories.

We believe we are just like everyone else, and so we start to believe that we are not special.

We go to our computers, trying to distract ourselves from our seemingly meaningless existence. The problem is that this only makes the situation worse: there are no meaningful relationships.

Burnout

Worker's constant internet access has rendered them fried, and eliminated any sense of "time-off". We're always connected and never truly isolated. To escape the world's stresses and excitement, we used go to work with friends or family.

We can now check on orders, receive emails, and complete reports even after we leave the office. We go to beautiful, remote places to rest and rejuvenate, but we don't forget to take photos and check emails. Other than the zip code, there is no change.

Slower Emotional Development

Children are more vulnerable to the dangers of digital media. While adolescents cherish solitude and independence in their lives, they have access to constant digital media.

A lot of codependency can be caused by constant contact between parents and friends. It can also lead to increased narcissism or a decline in empathy. Truth is, we are constantly de-sensitized by movies, music, social media and sensationalized information.

A digital detox forces you to confront real-world problems with real-world people, real-world emotions and real-world relationships. Without internet filters, we can begin to develop deeper emotional intelligence that can help us and others.

Physical Illnesses

Digital activity has been linked to several health issues. Inactivity may be the cause of some of these issues, such as heart disease and obesity. Others result from the physical actions of our devices.

People who spend too many hours in front of a computer screen are more likely than non-technological users to experience macular damage and worse vision. There has been an increase in neck, spine, and head injuries among heavy users.

Our posture is affected and we spend more time looking up than down. This causes misalignment and blurred vision.

An additional side effect is insomnia. It is experienced by those who cannot sleep due to their technology addiction. All of these issues are affected by stress, which is probably the most important. These symptoms not only can cause stress, they can also increase it.

How to do a Digital Detox... 6 steps!

Digital detoxes are a good place to start. It is nearly impossible to achieve this in today's climate without making a concerted effort. It may be impossible to live like the Amish for long periods of time, but we have some suggestions that will help you and your family spend less on technology and more time building healthy relationships.

Tip #1: Establish Ground Rules

Digital detox is something you need to discuss with your family when you aren't on a Google-free vacation. It's easier to be detached when you're on your own. Take the time to discuss what's best for everyone. It's important to set aside time for homework and email checking. Stick with it.

Your rules can be designed by choosing when, where, or how media will be used. Discuss the use of your gadgets and the times they are allowed. It is strongly recommended that you turn off your smartphone at night, put it in another room, wait at least one hour after getting up, before you start going online.

Instead of treating your device as an afterthought consider treating them as tools. We've already discussed how important it is to know the difference between work and pleasure time. Emails can wait when you are away from home or with friends. We guarantee that all emails and texts you have sent will still be accessible when your alarm goes off in the morning.

Tip 2: Schedule your Activities

Boredom is a common reason why people open their phones or turn on TVs. To avoid wasted tech time, it is crucial to plan activities. This could include anything from taking a trip to volunteer or cooking, as well as playing games, hiking, and crafting. It doesn't matter what, it doesn't matter how boring. You will have lots of fun activities to refer to when you need to play Candy Crush.

Planning activities can give you something to look ahead to, and can even lead to new traditions. Tuesdays might be for gaming or Wednesdays could be for bowling. The structure encourages meaningful connections between friends and family.

Tip #3: Keep your devices at home.

It may seem obvious while doing a digital cleanse, but many of us aren't able to do it. Our equipment is crucial for everything, including work, education and banking. However, it is necessary to spend some time away from technology.

There are many ways to achieve this. It can be more enjoyable, rewarding, and satisfying than you realize. Invite your friends or family to join you on a hike or camping vacation and ask them to all leave their phones at home. Gather together to share a free meal without your phone. Get maps and enjoy a good old-fashioned road trip.

While it may seem scary to abandon your smartphone and laptop, you will reap the many benefits. How many times have you been to dinner with friends without sending one text or snap? What about a vehicle ride you can take with your kids, but doesn't include Google Maps?

We know technology is changing rapidly and you won't be able to go back to the 1980s.

However, we can tell that spending more time with your devices will make it more enjoyable. A digital detox will help you gain a better perspective on how to limit your screen use every day.

Tip #4: Engage in Physical Activity

It has many benefits. One of these is the release and maintenance of endorphins. The stimulation of your body can help replace the dopamine that your device releases for hours each day. You can run, cycle, and swim while your gadgets are connected.

Exercise can also improve attention and memory and reduce stress and depression. It can also promote social bonds. It is essential to move to reduce the damage that electronics can do to your body.

Tip #5- Learn the Difference Between Healthy and Unhealthy Technology

There is a big difference between technology that is good and technology that is bad. It is normal to have your bank accounts, emails, maps, and music all on your phone. What about that downloaded game? What about social networking platforms? Are these things lifting you up or leading you down a rabbit tunnel of lost time, unfulfillment?

Let's do this: Get rid all the stuff you don't want. At least temporarily. For now, delete all apps related to games, social media and video streaming. You can suspend your social account for a short time. This may be a good way to get started with healthy tech habits.

While there are many benefits to using social media for watching shows and playing games, it is important to be clear. It's possible that you've spent too much time on these platforms. Instead of focusing on what is going wrong, think about what you are gaining.

Instead of sitting down in a restaurant trying desperately to find hashtags for that cute photo, you shot, get involved with the people around. While you may be rusty at the beginning, we promise that you'll be happier and better off if it continues.

Set a good example. Your children are totally immersed in digital life. It is almost impossible for them to imagine a life without cell phones and laptops. Have you ever seen children trying to use a Walkman? Children, even though they may pretend not to, depend on adults. If you keep work and home separate, it is possible to be a champion of family.

They need structure and look up to us as examples of how to behave. What happens when we keep checking our fantasy teams on Pinterest and uploading photos to Instagram all the time? They will, too. Plan some activities, set ground rules, and explain to your kids the importance of a detox. It will make you happy.

Tip #6

We don't need to be surrounded every minute of every day during a digital detox. It can actually be harmful and can make you return to your screen when you're alone.

This is especially important to young people, who may have never had the opportunity to be in total solitude without any technology. You are free to choose how you spend your time.

The most important thing is to be comfortable being alone with your thoughts. You can do a digital detox for as little as an hour each day to help you feel more connected with your emotions. This will allow you to be more compassionate and connect with others.

4 Ways To Prevent Relapse After Detox

Dopamine detox (and perhaps the most important) step in beating an addiction. Once you have completed this, you can begin your rewarding journey towards complete recovery.

A dopamine detox by itself is not enough to stop a person relapsing from treatment. Here are four ways to make sure you don't relapse after detox.

1. Use Your Support Network

To avoid relapse, your support network is a valuable resource. You shouldn't leave them behind, even when life gets difficult. You can rely on your friends and family to support you when you most need it.

Regular group meetings are a great way to get the support and guidance you need to avoid relapse.

2. A New Beginning

Relapse is much more common when the remnants from your past life are around you and constantly remind you about your addiction. Give yourself another chance for success by starting again. Take out all paraphernalia, dealers and apps from your home.

It may be necessary to change your phone number, or to relocate to another location in order to permanently end any harmful connections. For detox, it is essential to start over.

3. Maintain your routine

Keep yourself busy. Being productive and busy will make it easier to forget about the things that you have to fight with. Your desire to take addictive substances down may be reduced if positive changes are made in your life.

4. Stay Away from Triggers

Different people may experience different triggers that cause them to relapse. These triggers can be both emotional or environmental and are known to cause relapse in many people.

* Frustration Anxiety

* Depression

* Stress

People and places that are a reminder of what triggers the actions

When possible, avoid these trigger situations. It is impossible to escape negative emotions such as stress and despair. However, if you have a solid support network and can learn how you can divert yourself in useful ways, it will be easier to work through them and not relapse.

Chapter 6: Dopamine Detoxification Has Quantifiable Rewards

There are many backgrounds, psychology and physiology to consider, so the effect it has in your life is unique. You may find it the most remarkable thing you've ever done. Or, you might just do another thing.

Dopamine detox is likely to have a positive impact on all aspects of your daily life. Here are some examples.

Improved Financial Allocation. The old adage "time equals money" is quite true, especially when your time is charged by the hour (salespeople/contractors, etc.). You'll be able spend less and work more, but earn more.

Greater Time Management - It is common knowledge that you cannot do both at once. If you cut down on low-value tasks, you might be able to divert your time to something more worthwhile and valuable.

Motivation to succeed more - Although motivation is an intangible concept, its effects are tangible. You'll crave activities when there aren't as many stimuli. You'll feel bored. You can then channel that energy to something productive such as reading a novel or learning a new skill.

Higher Resonance to Life - This will allow life to take on greater significance. Your stimuli will be found "outside" of your body, so you will have to interact with others in order to obtain them. You will be interested to hear other people's stories. You'll want me to connect with you. You are a life citizen and will be interested to contribute value.

An increase in self-awareness is part of the dopamine detox. The detox involves removing any preconceived notions or beliefs that hinder us from exploring deeper and uncovering forgotten or overlooked parts of ourselves. It's impossible to be honest with yourself when you have less. This will help you understand yourself better and your motivations. It is hard work, but essential.

Enhances Creativity & Imagination - Your imagination is your only tool. Your imagination functions like a muscle. If you consume constantly, it's impossible to imagine. To be great, you must be alone with your thoughts. Your genius will amaze you. Give your mind space to relax. This is what the brain wants fast.

You can increase productivity and focus on long-term goals. Dopamine addiction will make you a failure.

People have made new habits and conditioned their brains so that they seek dopamine over long-term labor.

Your monkey brain is always looking for a reward, whether it's an Instagram notification or an updated phone message.

Everyone was taught to think in the immediate. This paradigm can be broken and you will be able conquer.

Everyone else is still standing. You are running a marathon. They may think they are faster, but in reality they are stuck on a treadmill. While you race to the finish line, your heart rate is soaring.

Break your Comfort Addiction-Dopamine addiction is a way to reduce the size of your comfort zone. To mask pain in today's pleasure-addicted culture, dopamine pills are being used.

Dopamine, a pharmaceutical, is one example. Dopamine is a drug. However, it has many more adverse effects than those listed in commercials.

Dopamine is used to prevent unpleasant events. Instead of confronting your own thoughts, boredom and anxiety head-on you retreat to your phone.

When was the last moment you didn't glance at your phone when you took a bite? Now, you are playing Candy Crush.

This could prove to be disastrous. Avoiding the situation only makes it worse. It's similar to letting a homeless person camp out at your door, afraid that you might say something. Then, all of sudden, he starts sleeping with you.

Dopamine gradually makes you more attached to comfort, which can weaken your ability to maintain discipline. You lose control. You lack the motivation to complete crucial activities.

You avoid undesirable experiences, as they do not trigger the same dopamine surges.

A dopamine fast is a long, tedious trek to freedom from this comfort prison.

It is important to remember that if everyone is conditioned for pleasure, they can endure long periods of suffering. Growing is not easy. A rallying cry is discomfort. A pleasure-obsessed society is boring. Their greatest achievement is their Fortnite score rather than their 100 years of Cathedrals.

A simple desire to escape discomfort can quickly turn into an addiction to comfort, which will eventually lock you in a comfortable prison.

A dopamine fast is a long, tedious trek to freedom from this comfort prison.

It is possible to have everything you want.

Dopamine Sensitivity. Rewire your Brain.

These demonic technologies can rewire your brain and cause you to be addicted to comfort.

Even if it doesn't feel like you are addicted, your brain is rewired. The reward seesaw has migrated towards the monkey brain more than towards the human brain as stated above.

Your brain knows that short-term goals are more important than long-term ones.

Each time you scroll through Instagram, while at work or school, you are creating new habit patterns in your brain.

You can train yourself to believe that distraction will result in a reward. There is no learning. Not skill development. Not making it.

You allow your thumb to take complete control. Our amazing opposable thumb evolved to conquer the globe. Now, it is a slave to the iPhone scroll. You are focusing too much on the wrong things, and you're looking for illusory results.

This dangerous technology will be gone the moment you grasp neuroplasticity. Every thought, action and thought that you make literally rewires your brain. This leads to subtle association behavior. It's almost like you took your car's dash apart and started plugging strange cables into each others. The radio goes into reverse the second you turn it on.

Chapter 7: Stop Procrastinating

Procrastination has been a common problem. Dickens described it as the "thief and time." But how can we overcome our procrastinating tendencies? It is possible to trick our brains into thinking that it is easier and more pleasant to do unpleasant things. You would be so much more productive if you never put off the things that you might do today.

Why do we procrastinate?

First, let's find out what is causing procrastination. It turns out there are biological reasons why procrastination happens. It's not all of our fault.

The problem arises from two brain areas that are in conflict: the limbic System (an older, unconscious brain area that includes our pleasure center) & the Pre-frontal Cortex (a more recent brain part which handles high-level task).

The limbic system focuses on what makes you feel happy. It naturally avoids unpleasant situations. It does not worry about the long-term or deadlines.

Your organizer, however, is your prefrontal cortex. This area is younger and less powerful than the rest of your brain. It loses to the limbic, which distributes dopamine for reward. In short, procrastination makes us feel happier (at least temporarily).

Dopamine Detox

A dopamine detox can be used to trick your brain into performing difficult tasks. This is a way to deprive your brain of dopamine over a long period. It is possible to find enjoyment in even boring, repetitive, or necessary tasks because your brain seeks stimulation.

Avoid dopamine-rich behaviors such as Netflix, internet surfing or phone surfing and sweet foods, alcohol, and other similar activities. Study after study has shown that disconnecting yourself from dopamine can increase mental attention and clarity.

A Timeline for Detail

You may be more likely to procrastinate if the project is difficult or large, or if you have only one deadline. It is easy to become overwhelmed by a single task, especially if you are painful.

Instead, try breaking down tasks into smaller steps with a tight deadline. You can build momentum by starting small. Instead of declaring that "I'll finish this presentation by next year," set a goal for two PowerPoint slides each day, and then cross them off as they are completed.

Collaboration with Others

It's easier to be lazy than to do anything if you're not held accountable or if no one is tracking your progress. Collaboration with someone you trust will help you to meet your deadlines if you are pressed for time.

You must be focused and meticulous, and not let your guard down. Your best office friend may not be the best antiprocrastination weapon. You can even use virtual coworking software to stay on task.

Be Free from Distractions

People procrastinate most because they are too busy. You can decrease their impact by having the discipline to resist these distractions (see: dopamine withdrawal). Place your phone in a different room.

Freedom and Forest are two examples of internet filtering tools. Turn off the phone or go to a quiet location away from other people and chatter. The more distractions you have, the easier it is to concentrate for long periods of time.

Reward Yourself

Psychologists refer to the habit loop as trigger, behavior, rewards. The job we don't like is the trigger that causes us to procrastinate. Avoiding that work is the default behavior. It feels good...to an extent. The reward is a temporary relief that, unfortunately, doesn't last for long. This system can be short-circuited by rewarding yourself each time you complete a task with a different and better reward. ......

Mindfulness

There is strong evidence that mindfulness can be used to reduce procrastination. There are several ways it does this. Mindfulness can help us get out of the negative feedback loop. It allows us connect to our emotions: curiosity and the pleasure in completing well-done work.

1

Dopamine, and the role that it plays

Dopamine acts as a neurotransmitter and transmits information from your brain into other organs. Dopamine can be both a great motivator and a hindrance to your success.

It's a key factor that drives you to reach greater heights and achieve your goals. That's why it's known as the chemical of creativity or desire. You can also see that it is one of the main drivers for romantic pursuits, earning the title of the chemical love. However, it is also the largest reason why we become addicted to substances or behaviors.

Dopamine has earned a name for itself as a chemical that inspires creativity, love and addiction. However, it also plays a crucial role in our physical, psychological, and spiritual well-being. Dopamine regulates many physiological functions in animal and human bodies. It is clear then that dopamine's presence or absence can dramatically affect an individual's well-being.

Let's start by taking a closer look at the mysterious chemical. We will see how it influences our lives and drives our behaviours.

What Is Dopamine Anyway?

Dopamine works as a neurotransmitter and acts as a chemical messenger between the neurons of your brain and your body. It is responsible for many physiological functions. More details will be provided.

Dopamine has a distinct effect on the brain, in addition to its health and mental benefits. Dopamine surges when your brain anticipates a reward. Doing a specific activity often triggers the feeling of reward-anticipation. Brain experience has shown that this particular activity is rewarding. Even though you're still engaging in the behavior, dopamine is released by the brain.

Your behavior is what triggers your brain. It is difficult to achieve the "high" that your brain desired when you have completed the behavior. If this happens, your brain and mood are affected by a lack of dopamine. As a result, you feel less satisfied than when you started.

Let's take one example to illustrate the point.

You may have experienced a time in your life when you craved that sugar rush just after the end of work. Let's imagine that you have a chocolate fudge cake waiting for you at your home and are just trying to reward yourself for all your hard work.

You're done with your work. You find nothing in the fridge. It's gone. Your spouse, siblings, children or anyone you live with just took the liberty to eat it.

I'm sure you are a responsible, mature adult who understands the importance of not crying when their sweets go missing. You wouldn't, however, cry in this circumstance - I know you would. Yet, why would something so trivial change our lives?

When we look at the situation, we will find the answer.

The result is that you have been fueling your dopamine throughout your day. The reward was eating the chocolate-covered cake, which is a treat that tastes like heaven. The only thing you could do was to go through the motions - which was far more difficult than it sounds. You were motivated by the idea that you would be generously recognized for your efforts if just you reached that goal.

The reward for your brain's dopamine level was supposed to be the hit. Your brain did not have enough dopamine to sustain the high anticipation for the dopamine hit. You did not get the dopamine boost from the reward. Your dopamine level also dropped below the normal baseline. You felt more disappointed and depressed than usual.

Let's say that you return home and find your chocolate cake. You bite into the cake and you are pleasantly surprised by the taste. However, you start to feel something wrong when you take the second one. Next you take the third, fourth and fifth bites. However, you are never able feel the same exhilaration that you felt with the first bite.

What does that mean? There's no way. It's okay to continue eating the entire cake even though it doesn't make you feel good.

This is the way dopamine works: it builds up in search of rewards. You don't feel satisfied when you get your reward. Instead, you crave more. It is also known as "the molecule of more".

The reinforcement phase, the final stage of the dopamine program, is now complete. Thanks to dopamine's influence, once your brain recognizes something as pleasurable, the cycle of "motivation-reward-reinforcement" keeps repeating in an endless loop.

How does Dopamine make you feel?

If you're talking about normal levels of dopamine, then the right dose will make your life perfect. You'll find yourself in a pleasant mood. You will be more productive, learn better, and plan better. The right dose of dopamine is physiologically necessary to feel alert, focused and motivated. Euphoria can be caused by a sudden dopamine boost.

Dopamine: What is its role?

Dopamine plays a key role in pleasure- and reward-centers, but it is much more than just being a drug whiz. It influences blood flow and sleep cycles, heart function, mood and stress response, as well as the kidney and kidney function.

However, dopamine does not act in all of these processes by itself. It only has the ability to exert its effects due to the support of other neurotransmitters like serotonin and adrenaline.

So, what exactly does dopamine (the neurotransmitter dopamine) do in our bodies. It plays the following roles:

1. Movement

Basal Ganglia is an area of the brain that controls movement. It can only function at maximum efficiency if it receives a certain amount dopamine. If the dopamine level is not optimal, then movement can become slow and uncoordinated. In contrast, excess dopamine can lead to unnecessary movements such repetitive tics or trembling.

2. Pleasure-seeking, Reward-Seeking Behavior

We've already covered how dopamine plays a major role in pleasure-seeking. It is responsible for causing the brain to seek pleasure and reward through sex, food, and drug abuse.

3. Memory

The importance of dopamine for memory is delicate. The prefrontal cortex is a crucial part of the brain that regulates and enhances working memory. Prefrontal cortex dopamine levels must be in balance. Any slight alteration in the dopamine level, either higher or lower affects memory greatly.

4. Attention

Dopamine helps with attention and focus. Dopamine has a dual effect on memory and attention. The prefrontal cortex controls our attention. Vision triggers the brain's dopamine response. This diverts attention away from one subject and focuses it on, but dopamine is responsible for what stays in the short term memory. It is believed that ADD can be caused by a lack of dopamine in this area.

5. Cognitive Function

Dopamine is crucial for cognitive function. Dopamine has many functions, including memory and attention. It also controls information flow between different brain centers. Dopamine deficiency will cause neurocognitive impairment, which will result in memory, attention, and problem solving skills being affected.

6. Pain Processing

Dopamine plays a crucial role in pain processing. Painful symptoms in neurodegenerative conditions like Parkinson's disease, such as Parkinson's disease, are magnified when dopamine levels fall.

7. Vomiting or Nausea

Dopamine is one the neurotransmitters that can control nausea or vomiting. Dopamine receptors are activated in chemotherapy patients by antiemetic drugs.

8. Secretion Prolactin

Prolactin regulates milk production in pregnancy and post-pregnancy. Dopamine is a major regulator that inhibits prolactin release.

9. Social Functioning

We'll be discussing this more in a bit. But dopamine plays a critical role in social functioning. People with low levels either of social anxiety or social fear have reduced dopamine use. However, those with high levels dopamine are often hyper-social and hypersexual.

Dopamine Abnormalities

Dopamine abnormalities can result in many problems, from mildly severe to extremely serious. Let's look at these conditions.

* Dopamine Deficiency

Dopamine deficiency often causes lethargy, and depression. You will notice an increase in moodiness, regardless of whether or not it is obvious. These symptoms can also occur

* Difficulty in Concentrating

* Low motivation and low enthusiasm

* A reduced alertness

* Lower motor skills like poor coordination and difficulty with movement

* Sleep problems are also known to reduce dopamine levels

More serious, reduced dopamine could cause serious mental or physical disorders. These include:

* Parkinson's disease

* Depression

* Dopamine transporter deficiency syndrome

* Dopamine Overload

When dopamine levels go up, you will feel an immediate rush of euphoria. That lasts for a while at least. You may go into overdrive when you take in more dopamine.

An abnormally high dose of dopamine can lead, in part, to severe mental disorders. This has been linked to schizophrenia and psychosis. Atypically high levels of dopamine can lead to:

* Hallucinations

* Mania

* Delusions

A high level of dopamine could also lead to:

* Schizophrenia

* Obesity

* Addiction

* Addiction

Dopamine in the normal pathway is secreted and reabsorbed by the brain. This delicate balance between dopamine and other chemicals is essential.

However, this balance is out of sync with addiction. Hard drugs like cocaine, amphetamines, can disrupt the dopamine pathway. Hard drugs such as cocaine, amphetamines, and nicotine can also cause disruptions in the dopamine-evoking cycle. We'll get into addiction more in the next chapter. But for now, we can understand how dopamine is affected by the substance chosen.

When this happens, the user begins to lose interest in all other things and becomes obsessed with that high feeling. Although behavioral addiction may not be as severe as alcohol and drug addiction, it is still a serious condition.

Evolution and Dopamine

It's not just us who have dopamine stored in our brains. Dopamine was discovered and first named in 1957. It is believed that dopamine's main functions are motor control, reward enforcement learning, and motor control. These are now the main functions of dopamine, in any living organism.

But, we now know that the role of dopamine in human behavior is complex. The higher dopamine levels that we have may be what has helped us reach the top of our social hierarchy.

According to the Proceedings of the National Academy of Sciences report, both humans and animals have higher levels of serotonin as well as neuropeptides. These neurotransmitters are responsible for cooperative behavior and social cues. The report did however highlight a major difference between humans and apes in dopamine levels. The dopamine levels in humans are significantly higher than the levels found in other animals.

We have more dopamine than apes which allows us to socialize in a complex manner. Scientists believe that the evolution pressure of complex social environments has led to higher levels of dopamine in the brain.

Digital Age: Dopamine overload

You're now finished.

Our digital age offers instant gratification for all the little things we do. Social media is an empire that's built around the goal of getting you hooked for more "like," comments, "share," and flashy content. Every piece of tech is intended to trigger excitement in your brain.

Does this sound like one those conspiracy theories? This is not what I am saying. It is Sean Parker, one the founding presidents Facebook.

Sean told the Guardian in an interview that Facebook was made to distract us, not connect us. He explained, "The thought process for Facebook was: 'How do you consume as much of the time and conscious awareness as possible?

Facebook architects decided to exploit a "vulnerability in human psychology". Everything on their app, from the comments you make to others' posts to the colors and layout, gives you a little dopamine.

Facebook can be deleted and all other social media apps as well as emails and video games that were available in the last 20 years of technology. Each of them was built around the same principle: instant dopamine hits. Giving up on them feels easy, but in reality it can be difficult.

Even in your offline activities, you have been programmed for instant gratification. Coffee is a way to instantly feel alert and focused. Smoking nicotine can also make you feel instant awake. Watching pornography makes you feel excited because it gives you an extreme edge that allows you to barely feel anything else. You shop for better images in anticipation of the floods of comments and likes that will come your way when you post new mirror selfies.

If you were to take a look at your life and consider what is driving it, you will see that the neurotransmitter dopamine is responsible. This tiny chemical is responsible both for your overwhelming anticipation and the feeling of underwhelming satisfaction when engaging in the behavior described above. It is, in short, the root cause behind all our behavioral and more serious addictions.

Understanding addiction is difficult without more information. We'll talk about this in the next chapter.

Here are some key takeaways

* Dopamine can be described as the chemical that creates desire, creativity or love.

* It also contains the molecule of additional, which allows you to pursue pleasure and reward-seeking behaviors.

* Dopamine plays an essential role in all major and minor physiological, psychological, and psychological functions.

* Any dopamine level change, whether it is higher or less, can lead to serious side effect.

* The majority of people believe that dopamine is a major cause of human development, as compared to other primates.

* Because technology triggers instant pleasure, nearly everyone suffers from dopamine overdose.

2

The Science of Addiction

In the past ten years, researchers have tried to understand the nature and effects of drug addiction. The science behind addiction is now more understood than ever. We are able to see the full range of substance abuse disorders, how their brains can be affected and how our behavior can change. Today we are more conscious of the compulsive nature drugs and that it is now a medical disorder. Scientists are working to discover genetic variations that might contribute to the development or progression of this disorder.

What is Addiction and How Does It Work?

Addiction, in simple terms, is the compulsive psychological/physiological need to take or use something until it harms you. Addiction is more than a dependency on drugs or alcohol. Addiction includes the inability to stop compulsive actions like gambling, eating and sex. Substance addiction may be considered a chronic condition. This can occur when certain medications are used, including prescription opioids.

There are two types: substance addiction or non-substance abuse. Substance abuse is the abusing of drugs with psychoactive effects. Non-substance abuse includes addiction to food, gambling, the internet and cell phones, as well as gaming and sex. The basic idea is that a person with addiction will continue to engage in the activity or the substance, regardless if it has any harmful effects.

According to American Society of Addiction Medical, addiction is a chronic, treatable medical condition that can be managed. It involves complex environments, life experiences and brain circuits as well as genetics. Add to that, many people with an addiction or substance abuse problem also have to deal with other psychological or physiological problems. Their biggest challenge is to recognize their need for help or making positive changes in life.

Often, people take up drug-taking out of a desire to do so. But as their bodies react to repeated doses, they become dependent and then are unable or unwilling to stop using the substance. When this happens, the person is a full-blown drug addict and can't control their cravings for their drug.

Differentiating between drug misuse and addiction

These two terms often get confused and are mistakenly thought to describe the same thing. Drug misuse refers a misusing of a substance at high levels or using it in an unsuitable manner that can lead to health or social issues. Although it sounds similar to addiction, this is not the same thing.

The problem of addiction is not necessarily a result of misuse. One example is that some people can drink alcohol very heavily and feel both the harmful effects and the euphoric effects. This does not necessarily mean they have an addiction problem.

Addiction Symptoms & Withdrawal Effects

Poor performance in work or problems with relationships are two of the most obvious indicators that someone is struggling with an addiction. Addicts tend to lash out at those around them, which can lead to a problem of self-deprecating behavior. An addiction sign is a decreased performance in school or difficulties with participation in activities. Addicts will be unable to stop using the substance even if they have health or personal issues. You will experience extreme fatigue, loss of energy and changes in your appearance. The person experiencing this problem will act defensively, refuse to believe that there is anything wrong and be aggressive when confronted.

The withdrawal symptoms, which are the absence of the substance or indulging in it, is another classic sign of an addiction problem. These withdrawal symptoms can be described as a string of strong symptoms that point to a person's physical dependency on the substance. These withdrawal symptoms can often be observed in cases of abrupt discontinuation of an abuse substance (and in some cases may even prove fatal).

Why Do People Use Drugs?

Many factors can lead to an addiction. You may feel pleasure at first, but then you start to notice changes in your mental and physical state. This creates an unconscious desire to experience the same euphoria again. These substances can become addictive and people feel a strong urge to continue using them. Gambling has a similar psychological effect. Gamblers experience a heightened sense of pleasure when they win. This is followed by a need to retry. This becomes a compulsive behaviour that is hard to quit.

Ironically, people's drug-taking behaviors often begin as an attempt at taking control of their lives, but it eventually takes that control away. At first, substance abuse appears to be a promising solution. However, it soon becomes a frustrating and debilitating problem. It can also be a way to feel mature, experiment or relax. This last reason is more common among teenagers and young adults.

Simply stated, the substance triggers certain neurological pathways in your brain, generating a feeling called euphoria. The feeling of euphoria fades after a while. To experience the same intensity, you need to take more. This leads to a problem with the brain that can become a chronic problem. It also causes a compulsive disorder that affects one's physical and mental health.

Many reasons can cause strong emotional stress in a person. One reason could be the loss of a loved one, drastic changes in financial circumstances, divorce, or chronic health problems. Many people turn to drugs to manage emotional distress or improve their focus and endurance. Additionally, drug abuse can be caused by mental illness, trauma or an attitude toward society.

Different Usage Types

Understanding addiction science is essential. This includes learning about the factors and reasons that lead to drug misuse. This is because different situations could lead to a different frequency of drug abuse. A variety of factors can play a significant role in the addiction issue, including both intrinsic and extrinsic. These categories should not be viewed as absolutes. Many drug users will move from one type to the next. Below are six general categories that cover the reasons drug users use drugs.

1. Experimental Causes: A person may use a drug or substance just out of curiosity. In time, curiosity turns into an obsession and a

persistent habit that adversely affects their well being.

2. Situational Factors - A person might start using a substance when they are dealing with situational factors such as peer pressure, stress, or feeling shy.

3. Recreational Use: Here, the user is using the substance to have fun, relax, or to elevate their mood.

4. Excessive Bingeing: The drug user might begin to consume a high amount of the drug temporarily. Over time, however, this may become a regular behavior.

5. Therapeutic Use of the Drug: Although some people use the drug to treat a medical condition, it could also be used for therapeutic purposes.

6. Dependent Usage: When a person is addicted and has been using the substance for a prolonged period of time. This is when the individual feels compelled to use the

substance again to feel normal, and to avoid withdrawal.

Common Triggers to Addiction

Before diving into the common triggers we need to first understand what a trigger actually is.

So what exactly is a trigger'? The APA dictionary, 2019, defines a trigger as a stimulus that elicits a response. Triggers can be considered to be an important contributor to the initiation of a craving for a drug or substance. This will result in increased addiction behavior. These triggers and external stimuli can often push an individual to compulsive drug consumption. They may also lead to relapse following a period or voluntary abstinence.

Although there are many reasons people may start using drugs for psychological, physiological, and other reasons, some environmental triggers or biological factors can increase the risk of developing an addiction.

Below we'll discuss some of the causes that could trigger or contribute towards an increase in addiction becoming chronic.

1. Social Acceptability

Alcoholism is accepted socially and is often celebrated in our society. People often drink freely at parties and are unaware of the negative consequences. The primary reason people start to consume alcohol is social gratification. The collective cultural consciousness at parties often places alcohol front and center. It is an accepted symbol, and many people believe they wouldn't fit in without a glass of wine.

2. Peer Pressure

Peer pressure is something we all deal with, especially in our younger years. People around us start to validate us by doing many things. In return, we act the same way they do. Peer pressure often causes people to change their personalities to fit in with the group and avoid being seen as an outsider. This is often combined with the desire for approval and to be considered 'cool.

3. The grief of losing a loved-one

A sudden loss of a loved is devastating and can cause depression. Recovering from trauma like this is not an easy process for everyone. Some people are able to heal quickly, and then go back to their regular lives. Others may need to struggle for many years. This group is at high risk of getting addicted to drugs to try and find relief.

4. Moving through the Loss Of A Relationship

People can also become addicted to drugs after a breakup or divorce, particularly if they don't have enough support. This not only impacts the self-confidence, but also has consequences for other relationships. They use drugs to help them cope with all the negative events in their lives.

5. You are struggling with a psychological illness

Psychological illnesses can be difficult to manage. When people attempt to deal with them on their own, it often leads to a lot of frustration. This multifaceted condition can have different triggers. Some people will attempt to justify their psychological problems while others turn to drugs and alcohol in an effort for relief.

6. Escape from Life-Stressors

All of us know that life can be difficult. When someone enters the adult stage of their lives, they must learn how to balance work and home, pay regular expenses, manage relationships, and so on. Not everyone is mentally ready to deal with these issues. Some will choose drug abuse as a way to find some peace.

7. Environmental Influences

People who have been raised in an environment of poverty, crime and drug use are at high risk of using drugs or alcohol. Many of these people see drugs and alcohol as their natural way of living. They have never seen anything better, and it is continued.

8. Inability or unwillingness to meet family demands

Most people are capable of handling increasing demands from their families as they grow. For ambitious young mothers, it can be hard to make the transition from one phase to another, especially if they aren't able to continue their careers.

9. Performance Enhancement or Focus

Some drugs have properties that enhance performance for a brief time. People who use these drugs feel they have an ability to improve their focus, memory, cognition, as well as their concentration. They become an addiction over time as the drug's effects decrease.

10. Escaping Boredom

Boredom is another trigger for drug addiction. People with less responsibilities and more income are more likely to use drugs to alleviate boredom. This is their way of passing the time.

11. You can have fun getting "high"

Most drug addicts believe that they took up the habit as an experiment. Dopamine, which is a neurotransmitter linked to pleasure and feelings of pleasure, is released in most drugs. They continue taking the same drug until they feel the same euphoria.

Science of Addiction & Dopamine

It is a common misconception that those who take drugs are morally and psychologically weak enough to succumb to addiction. Drug addiction is a complicated condition and requires professional support. The brain's neurological responses to drugs or other drugs can be so severe that it is difficult for people to quit. Different drugs will cause different brain responses.

1. These drugs are often similar to the brain's natural neurotransmitters. The brain responds to these drugs in a similar way to heroin and marijuana. When the drug attaches at the receptor sites, it activates corresponding neurons. Then, they send exaggerated neural messages to CNS (central nerve system).

2. The drug of abuse, particularly methamphetamine or cocaine, floods our reward circuit, leading to an excessive release of dopamine, which is linked to the brain's reward system. Dopamine, which is a potent neurotransmitter, also regulates cognition. It can also control movement, emotion, cognition, and motivation. Dopamine stimulates the brain to produce a sudden rush of dopamine. This can lead to an overpowering reinforcement of addictive behaviors. This creates a stronger connection between pleasure and use of the particular drug. Increases in dopamine levels that are sudden and dramatic can cause our brains' compulsive search for the substance or drug.

3. Also, drugs and alcohol can disrupt our brain's neurochemical systems and neural circuits. These circuits are responsible for executive cognitive functions like memory, stress, learning, behavior control and judgment. Once a person is aware of their life-threatening effects, it can be very difficult to quit using these drugs.

4.

What Happens When Someone Takes A Drug?

Each person has a neuronal reward system that controls the reinforcement of their behaviors. The reward system should function properly to motivate the person's behavior. It regulates our natural behaviors by activating the reward system at a normal frequency. Addiction is a different story. The reward circuit plays a role in drug-taking because of the pleasure it provides. This can lead to an increased dependence on drugs or harmful substances.

This happens when the reward circuit is overstimulated, leading to physical dependence.

The brain's neural networks change and adapt to new situations as the drug user continues to take the drug. They also reduce the reward circuit cells ability to respond. This decreases the overall feeling of being "high" as the drug addict experienced when they first tried it. This is called 'tolerance'. Users may take more of the substance to get the same sensation.

These neural adaptations would lead to a gradual decrease in pleasure from the drug/substance of abuse. Many adverse physiological symptoms, also known as withdrawal symptoms, can result from abruptly stopping the use or taking away the substance.

Anticipation & Preoccupation

The neural changes that are caused by continuous use of the addictive drug can often lead to obsession or obsessive anticipating. A drug user may experience intense cravings as addictive substances exert a stronghold over their brain and can alter brain circuitry (also known to be 'conditioned reinforcement'). This impacts their ability to make informed decisions and can lead to a decline in their ability for decision-making.

Unfortunately, every time a user takes the drug, their conditioned reinforcements increase. It becomes increasingly difficult for users to abstain. This vicious cycle is extremely difficult for drug users.

Why is it that some people are more vulnerable than others?

There are many factors which increase the chance of developing an addictive problem. This means that people with more addiction risk than others are at greater risk. However, certain individuals may be at greater risk because of biology, environmental, and developmental factors.

Research suggests that around 40% to 60% are at risk for developing an addictive condition due to their genetic makeup. This includes epigenetics (effects environmental factors have on our genetic expression) as well as the family history. The risk of addiction is increased if someone has been diagnosed having a behavior disorder like anxiety or depressive symptoms.

An addiction is defined as a lifelong dependence on a substance, activity or drug. It requires professional treatment. Addicts may have difficulties abstaining or engaging in harmful behavior. Careful interventions and treatment are needed.

3

Dopamine Addiction - The Most Common

As we saw in the previous chapter, dopamine (a neurotransmitter which affects our sense of pleasure) is the chemical released in an active addict. The dopamine rush becomes a craving in our brains and we are unable to stop searching for it. Withdrawal symptoms are a common reaction for addicts when they stop using a substance that isn't considered a drug.

Some people will not become addicted to these activities. Dopamine addictions are very dangerous for those who are genetically, or psychologically, susceptible. This chapter will examine the most prevalent dopamine addictions. We'll discuss how they are manifested, detox timelines, and tips for beating them.

Sugar Detox

Your brain releases dopamine as a response to sugary sweets, just like if you ingested heroin. Sugar addiction can result in a dopamine rush that can make it addictive. Many people can't resist the temptation to continue eating sweets. Sugar addiction is one among the most harmful dopamine addictive behaviors. Because sugar is hidden within many processed foods and is not considered a substance that should be taken seriously, detoxing from sugar addiction can be challenging.

Sugar Addiction: The Dangers

Sugar can cause obesity, type II diabetes, heart disease and cancer. Too much sugar can also lead to mood swings as well anxiety and depression. Sugar plays a significant role in this epidemic, with more than two thirds of Americans being overweight or obese. Sugar consumption is linked to the following health risks:

* Obesity. Have you ever tried to stop eating sweets until your bag is full? Does this sound familiar? You may be familiar with this: The more sugar you eat, the more you will eat and the more likely you are to be overweight or obese. Sugar is high in empty calories, so sugary foods are easy to overeat.

* Type 2 diabetes: Sugar causes blood sugar to spike and can eventually lead to type 2. Diabetes is a serious condition that can lead to blindness, heart disease and stroke.

* Heart Disease: High sugar intake can increase your risk for heart disease. It raises bad cholesterol levels and triglycerides. It can also increase inflammation, which is a significant risk factor for developing heart disease.

* Cancer: While sugar is not proven to cause cancer, some believe it can fuel tumor growth and feed cancer cells. It has been linked with many different types of cancer, including colon cancer, breast cancer and pancreatic carcinoma.

* Mood swings - Sugar can cause mood swings, anxiety, depression. Hypoglycemia may also occur. This is where you feel dizziness and shakiness.

* Other Health Problems - Sugar can also lead to headaches, tooth decay and arthritis.

Sugar addiction can lead you to crave sweet foods, increase weight, mood swings and problems with concentration and concentration. You may feel fatigued, irritable or have difficulty sleeping. You may experience nausea, vomiting, or headaches when you detox from sugar addiction. Some people experience flu-like symptoms like fever, chills or body aches.

How Sugar Addiction is manifested

Sugar addiction can come in many forms. Some people are addicted to sugar, while others get addicted to the comfort foods. Sometimes, people develop a sugar addiction to antidepressants or birth control pills. It begins with just a little bit of sugar daily, but it becomes more frequent over time. They could eventually be consuming so much sugar, it can cause damage to their health.

Children are especially susceptible to sugar addiction because their brains are still in development. According to the American Academy of Pediatrics (AAP), children aged 2-19 should not consume more sugar than 25 grams daily. That's six teaspoons. The American Heart Association recommends a daily intake of no more sugar than six teaspoons for women and nine for men for adults.

How to Get Over Sugar Addiction

While it may seem difficult to get rid of sugar, it is possible. You can get help for sugar addiction.

* Eliminate processed foods. These foods are high in sugar and should be avoided. Instead, eat whole, unprocessed meals.

Healthy eating habits are key to beating sugar addiction. You should eat plenty of fruits and vegetables and lean protein.

* Get Enough Sleep. To overcome sugar addiction, it is important to get enough sleep. If you are healthy, it is less likely that you will crave sugar.

* Exercise: Regular exercise can help curb your desire to eat sugary or unhealthy foods. It can also help improve moods and energy levels which can help you stay motivated and stick to your new health and diet.

* Get support Talk to them about what you want and ask them to help. You might even be able to find support groups in your community.

Sugar Detox: Duration

Detoxing from sugar addiction can take anywhere between a few days and a few months. It all depends upon how much sugar and how addicted. It's important to be patient and only take one step at the time. Stay focused and motivated to overcome your addiction.

Porn Detox

An unhealthy obsession with pornography online is more serious than you might think. It's a real addictive behavior, just as any other. You don't have control over how much, when, or for how long. It consumes your thoughts so much that you feel the need to constantly think about it. It causes you to lose your interpersonal relationships. It reduces your social life as well as your ability to interact with other people in real-life. Even worse, it makes it harder to be intimate and loving with another person.

The Dangers and Benefits of Porn

It can negatively impact your physical health. It makes it difficult to stop using it. However, it can make it easier to use (though you may feel worse - your brain tricks you into believing otherwise). It will affect your work performance. It is a major cause of procrastination. It takes away time that could be spent doing more important things.

Porn addiction can make you less spiritual and cause you to lose your ability to love, appreciate, and accept beauty and others. It can make you see people as objects, and not fellow human beings. Although there are many negative consequences of porn, it can also cause erectile dysfunction. Many people cannot seem to quit porn despite the fact that it is damaging their relationships, productivity, and health.

The symptoms

Obsessive sexual behavior is the hallmark of sexual addiction, despite the numerous negative consequences. Although there is no specific diagnosis for sexual addiction (or any other disorder), clinicians and researchers have tried to diagnose the disorder using criteria drawn from chemical dependency literature. These symptoms include preoccupations with fantasies, urges, or behaviors sexually, as well as an inability to control the impulses.

Porn Addiction? Get rid of it!

First, learn about sexual addiction. Read relevant articles and books. The concept of porn addiction is a new one for many people. Knowing that there are resources available will be a great help and a boost to your confidence. The more you learn about porn addiction, then the better. The less power you have over something, the better. There is no miracle cure. It will take energy, commitment, and time to make it happen. These guidelines can be helpful:

* Identify your triggers. It will be easier to manage addictive behaviors if you are aware of what triggers them.

* Be aware and present in your emotions. This will allow you to learn more about your own personality and help you identify what is causing you addiction.

* Reach out to others who have experienced porn addiction. These groups are particularly helpful.

* Maintain a healthy lifestyle, including eating well, staying active, getting enough sleep, and managing your stress levels.

* Learn new coping strategies, such as mindfulness and yoga.

Video Games Detox

Videogame addiction can be described as a behavioral addiction that leads to an obsession-compulsive urge to play videogames. Videogame addicts spend hours playing videogames every day, which can have devastating effects on their relationships, careers, and schools. Video game addiction has become a serious problem. According to the National Center for Biotechnology Information (NCBI), video games are addictive for 9 percent of Americans and 6 percent of Americans.

It is relatively new and we still have much to learn about widespread video gaming addiction. Teenagers are most vulnerable to this addiction. According to a University of Texas at Austin study, 88% of American teenagers use video games. Half of those who play video game for more than three hours per day are video gamers.

The Consequences of Addiction to Video Games

Video games addiction can lead to many problems. People addicted to video gaming may be unable or unwilling to work, study, or maintain a healthy relationship. People who play video games for extended periods of time may develop health problems like carpal tunnel syndrome and poor vision. Video gaming addiction can cause more harm than the individual.

Excessive gaming can lead a person to become isolated and even violent. It is not clear if this addiction has serious consequences, but there is much that we still don't know. There is hope for addicts to video games. There are many treatment options to help overcome addiction.

The following symptoms can be experienced by people addicted to video gaming:

* Obsessive Thoughts. Addicts often think about video games all the time. It is possible for them to feel that they cannot concentrate on any other task until they have played.

* Tolerance. Some people who are addicted to video games may need longer playing times in order to feel the same satisfaction.

* Withdrawal - Addicts will experience withdrawal symptoms if it isn't possible to play. This happens just like other addicts. These symptoms could include anxiety and irritability as well as bad temper and depression.

* Loss Interest in Other Activities. Those who are addicted to video gaming may lose interest other activities, like time with friends or going the gym.

* Consistent Use: Some video game addicts can play video games for hours, sometimes without eating and even sleeping.

How Video Game Addiction Develops

The way that video game addiction manifests can vary from one person to the next. One person may be more likely than another to spend hours playing video games alone, or to become aggressive or violent. Videogame addiction can manifest itself in many ways.

For some, video game addiction can have devastating consequences. Due to their gaming addiction, they could lose their jobs or fall behind in school work. A lot of video gaming can lead to health problems such as back pain, carpal tunnel syndrome or poor vision.

Some withdrawal symptoms, like depression and anxiety, can be common with many addictions. Others, like aggression and anxiety, can be specific to videogame addiction. If you want to get rid of videogame addiction, it is crucial to understand what symptoms each person experiences. This will help you to understand the problem and get treatment.

Video Game Addiction - Detox

It is not possible to detox from your addiction to video games in a single way. Some may require treatment at an inpatient center while others may be able and able to manage their addiction on their own. The process of detox will vary depending upon the individual and their addiction. There are a few things that can be helpful during detox from videogame addiction.

* Seek Professional Assistance: Expert help is essential during detox. You need the support to overcome your addiction.

* Remove All Access to Video Games. Although it may seem obvious, this is an important step. Get rid of any video games or consoles that allow you to play video game.

* Replace Video Games With Other Activities: Find other ways to fill your time that don't involve technology. This could be walking, reading or watching movies. It can also include spending time with friends.

* Make a New Routine. Take your time while you detox from gaming addiction. It is important to stop using video gaming as a tool.

* Be patient. It is not easy to detox from an addiction. Be patient with your self and realize that you can overcome this addiction.

Timeframe for detoxing from Video Game Addiction

There are many factors that affect the time taken to kick your video game addiction. Some people can recover in a matter of weeks, while others might need to detox for several months. Success will depend on many factors including the severity and support received from family and friends. It will take some time and effort to complete the detox process. Be positive even if your addiction doesn't disappear overnight. You can overcome your video game addiction with the right help and support

Smartphone addiction

Smartphones are an integral part our lives. However, they can also be addicting like any other thing. Most people will agree that smartphones have become too dependent on them, and they are being used for things that we shouldn't. This has made it commonplace to constantly check our phones, even when we are with people.

Even if we're not on our phones, we think about them. We can't help but keep checking our phones for new messages, notifications, and emails. When we aren't using our phones, it makes us feel anxious and helpless. This is the definition of addiction.

Smartphone addiction is not a recognized disorder but it is a problem. This problem will only continue to grow as people become more dependent on their phones.

Reality of Smartphone Addiction

Most people don't believe they are addicted to their smartphone. The truth is that many of our smartphones are addictive. Smartphone addiction can lead to serious health problems that must not be ignored. These are just a few of the many dangers that smartphone addiction poses.

* Less Productivity: Our productivity is affected by our constant checking of our phones. Our productivity suffers because we're constantly distracted.

* Increased stress: We check our phones constantly for new notifications. Anxiety is caused by the constant desire to be connected.

* Damaged Relationships This can be detrimental to your relationships.

* Negative effects on Mental Health: Smartphones may have negative consequences for our mental well-being. There are many things that can make us feel anxious, depressed, or even psychotic.

* Health Problems: The use of smartphones can also pose a threat to your physical health. As we are not getting enough sleep, don't exercise enough and are constantly stressed, we're more likely than ever to get sick.

* Driving While distracted by smartphones: Smartphones can make driving dangerous. We are more likely not to pay attention to traffic and to cause accidents.

How Smartphone Addiction Develops

Smartphone addiction displays in different ways for different people. One sign of an addiction to smartphones is the time they spend using them. It is possible for someone to spend hours on their phone and not realise how much time has passed. Other people may experience a subtler addiction. It may be that they only check their phone once an hour but the urge to do so is overwhelming.

There are many other ways that people use smartphones. Some use their phones for communication with loved ones, while others use them for entertainment. Some people use smartphones to escape from real life. These people feel that smartphones provide comfort and escape.

How to Get Rid of Smartphone Addiction

When you realize you are addicted to your smartphone, you need to act. Here are some steps you should take to get rid of your addiction.

* Make Changes in Your Phone Habits. Be more aware of how your phone is used. Reduce the amount of time that you spend on it and be more deliberate about how you use it.

* Disconnect Your Phone: A second way to end your addiction to your phone is to turn off your notifications and disconnect. This involves turning off all notifications, putting the phone away, and making sure you don't use it while you're out with friends.

* Look for Other Connections: You shouldn't rely solely on your phone. Find other ways to connect with your family and friends. Spend time talking with them in person or check out a messaging application that allows group chats.

* Find Other Ways To Pass the Time: If the only thing you do is use your phone to get through the day, look for other options. Go for a walk or to a movie.

* Get Enough Sleep. One of the best strategies to defeat smartphone addiction is to get enough rest. When you are tired, you are more likely to reach out for your phone.

* Seek Professional Assistance: If your addiction isn't solvable on your own, professional help may be needed. Many therapists offer help with smartphone addiction.

Detoxification from Drug and Alcohol

It can be challenging to detox from drugs and alcohol. It can be dangerous and it is crucial to seek professional help. It can be fatal, and it is not like other addictions. Your body goes through withdrawal when you have finished with detoxing from drugs and alcohol. You might experience various symptoms, some of them potentially dangerous.

The detox process takes about two weeks. Others can take up six months. For some, however, the detox process may take longer. The duration of your detox depends on the substance that you are addicted to, and how long you have been using it. It is difficult to manage detox on your terms and it is not recommended. A professional can keep an eye on your progress and ensure you are safe. They can also help you with guidance and support.

How Drug and Alcohol Addictions Are Manifested

You can see different signs of alcohol and drug addiction. Some people become dependent on alcohol or drugs after using them for a limited time. Some people may turn to drugs and alcohol to help with anxiety or stress. Addiction to drugs or alcohol can lead to a lifelong addiction.

According to the National Institute on Drug Abuse, addiction can be described as a "chronic, irrelapsing brain disease." That means you need to manage it throughout your life. Although there is no cure of addiction, there are treatment options that can help manage your condition.

Addiction to Drugs and Alcohol

Different people may have different symptoms. There are some symptoms you may notice that can be indicative of drug and alcohol addiction.

* Tolerance means you can tolerate more of the drug/alcohol in order to get the same effect.

* Withdrawal - When you stop using drugs and alcohol, withdrawal symptoms will occur.

* Craving: You will still crave the drug or drink, even if it has negative consequences in your life.

* Loss Of Control: You'll have no control over your alcohol and drugs use, and will not be able to stop using them.

* Social withdrawal: You'll stop talking to your friends and family.

* Financial Problems. Your addiction could lead to financial problems.

* Legal Problems

* Emotional Issues: You might experience anxiety, depression, and paranoia.

* Physical Problems. Your addiction could lead to a host of physical problems.

How to detox from alcohol and drugs

There are many types and forms of drug or alcohol addiction. Some may be addicted prescription drugs while others may be addicted street drugs. Some people might be addicted to alcohol while others may be addicted marijuana. To overcome alcohol and drug addiction can be a very difficult disease. But with the help and guidance of a professional as well as a 12 step program you can manage your addiction to live a healthy lifestyle. Here are some steps to help you detoxify from drugs and alcohol.

Talk to Your Doctor. Discuss with your doctor the best way to detox. They might recommend a specific detox program for you, or may prescribe medication to help you detox.

* Participate in a Detox Program. The best program for you and your needs is the one that you choose.

* Safe Detoxification: Make sure your detox program is staffed by professionals who can track your progress and assure your safety.

* Do it slowly: You shouldn't detox from drugs and alcohol too quickly. Rapid detoxing can be dangerous and could lead to relapse. To be safe, take your time and detox slowly.

* Get professional help: This is the best way to get professional support during and after detox. A professional can help you manage your addiction.

Detox can last anywhere from a few hours to several weeks, depending on the type and severity of your drug or alcohol addiction. You should follow the advice of your doctor to ensure a safe detox.

Gambling Detox

Gambling addiction is also known as pathological gambling. It involves gambling compulsively. You might feel the need to gamble more, even though you realize the harmful effects it has on your life. Gambling addiction has led to the loss of homes, jobs, families, and even their homes.

According to the National Council on Problem Gambling (NCPG), there are two million problem gamblers across the United States. While gambling addiction isn't as widely discussed as addictions to drugs and alcohol, it can have devastating consequences. Gambling addiction can cause financial, legal and emotional problems.

Gambling Addiction is a real problem

Gambling addiction may manifest in many different ways. Some people gamble compulsively while others only gamble when they have the chance. Some gamble just for fun while others are trying to escape their problems. Gambling addiction can cause serious problems in your life. Here are the most frequent symptoms:

* Gambling More Than You Can Afford: You'll bet more than what you can afford, even though it may mean taking out loans and going into debt.

* Losing control: You will lose your ability to control your gambling and be unable stop playing, even if it's something you really want.

* Gambling despite Negative Repercussions: You will gamble regardless of the negative impact it is having on your life.

* Gambling to Escape from Problems: To escape your problems, boredom, or stress, you'll bet on gambling.

* Telling lies to cover gambling: You will tell your family and friends to cover up your gambling.

* Feeling anxious/depressed: This could be due to gambling addiction.

How to get out of a Gambling Addiction

You need professional help in order to overcome gambling addiction. There are many treatments and programs available to treat pathological gambling. Here are some of these most popular treatments:

* Cognitive-Behavioral Treatment: This type therapy can help you change your gambling mindset and behavior. You will meet with a counselor regularly to discuss your addiction, and help you overcome it. The therapist may give you homework assignments to assist you in changing your thoughts or behaviors.

* Group Therapy - This is a type therapy in which you meet with people who are also struggling with addiction. You can share your experiences with them and learn from them.

* Medication - There are medications that can help you overcome your gambling addiction. These medications can reduce your desire and urge to gamble. Naltrexone is most commonly prescribed for gambling addiction.

* Rehabilitation: A type of treatment that requires you to live in a rehabilitation center for a certain amount of time. This type can be very helpful for those suffering from severe gambling addiction. The rehab center can provide counseling and therapy to assist you in overcoming your gambling addiction.

* Online Self Help Forums: These forums offer self-help for gambling addicts. These groups let you share your experiences with people suffering from the same addiction. They are a great way to get advice and support without having to leave your home.

One type of impulse control disorder is pathological gambling. It affects millions worldwide. It is still considered a gambling addiction. However, it can be just like any other addiction. Gambling addiction can have severe consequences and cause great harm to your health. Gambling addiction can make it difficult to overcome. But, you can get help from professionals. Look for a program that is right for you and make sure to stick with it. To find out more, contact your local addiction centre.

Here are some key takeaways

Dopamine can be involved with many different addictions. However, this chapter focuses on some of the most prevalent dopamine addictions. Here's a list of some key points to remember about this chapter.

* Dopamine (a neurotransmitter) is linked to pleasure and reward.

* Dopamine can lead to addiction because it provides an addictive rush of pleasure.

* The most common dopamine-related addictions are to sugar, porn (video games), gambling, drugs, alcohol, and other substances.

* If you want to get rid of sugar addiction, replace sugary foods with healthy ones and watch your sugar intake.

* You can detox from porn addict by avoiding watching porn. Seek professional help.

* To get rid of your addiction to video gaming, reduce the time spent on them and substitute other activities.

* Limit your smartphone use to detox from smartphone addiction.

* Get professional help and a detox program to get rid of your drug and alcohol addiction.

* Seek professional help and participate in a detox program to get rid of gambling addiction.

* The most popular treatments for dopamine addiction are cognitive-behavioral treatment, group therapy (medication, rehabilitation, and self-help online forums).

Talk to a licensed professional if you're struggling with dopamine dependence. There are many programs and treatments for dopamine addiction. Stick with the program that works best for you. It will be a long and difficult road, but it will pay off in the end.

4

Dopamine Fasting, Diets

Dopamine fasting is something that has become a popular topic in the last few decades. Dopamine Fasting is a practice that prevents you from enjoying pleasure-based activities such as eating, drinking, and using social media. The idea is that your brain will be able to manage your impulses better by temporarily avoiding food and drink.

The New York Times was one of the most prominent outlets to cover this fad. But experts have sharply condemned it as lacking any scientific basis.

However, what if it's something you still want to try? What does dopamine-fasting mean for your diet

There are many methods that you can use to stop your dopamine addiction. These include dopamine fasting as well as dopamine diets. This chapter will first explain what dopaminefasting is, then discuss the benefits. This chapter will also talk about how to adjust your nutrition for dopamine-fasting and whether or not it is worth the effort. Last but not least, we'll be looking at some of the most common dopamine fasting diets and their differences.

What is Dopamine Fasting, and how can it help you?

Sometimes, addiction to certain foods is just as dangerous as addiction to drugs or alcohol. The most common culprits are sugar, salt, and processed food. Although it can be hard to stop an addiction, the dopamine fast may help.

Dopamine Fasting is a way to stop your addiction to dopamine. It limits the amount of stimulants that trigger dopamine. This practice may also be without social media, technology, or food.

Dopamine fasting may help reduce brain dependence upon external sources. It is known to improve motivation and creativity as well as empathy and overall outlook.

A "dopamine fast," as it is commonly known, seems impossible for most people. It would be something that only a monk could do. Dopamine, the chemical responsible for motivation and pleasure, is constantly being released by our brains.

It might seem like this is a good thing. But, according to researchers, our society is constantly being bombarded with stimuli that are enjoyable. Many people find themselves craving these things more often than they should. This can cause obesity and addiction.

While you can't stop dopamine from being released by your brain, fasting allows you to restrict the things that cause it. Although there is nothing wrong with these things, it can be very difficult to let go of them when they become a habit. This is where dopamine fasting steps in.

How to Adjust Nutrition For Dopamine Fasting

There is no perfect diet for dopamine-fasting. You can adapt your nutrition to make the fast more effective.

1. Reduce Your intake of sugar, processed food, and caffeine

Dopamine production is stimulated by caffeine, processed foods, sugar, as well as stimulants like caffeine. These foods should be avoided while you fast. Be sure to read labels carefully and stay away from sugar, high fructose corn sirup, artificial sweeteners and other harmful ingredients. The same applies to caffeine. Dopamine fasting means that you should avoid caffeine and tea. You can make a plan about what you'll eat and how much.

2. More Whole Foods

Whole foods are healthier than processed foods, and they contain more nutrients. They also have a lower glucosemic index which means that they won't cause blood sugar spikes. You should eat at least 50% whole foods, which means that you include whole grains, fruits, vegetables and lean meats in your diet. By paying more attention to how your body feels after eating certain foods, you can also eat mindfully. If you feel happy after eating a food, then it is likely that it's a good choice to dopamine fasting.

3. Drink plenty of fluids

Fluids are important as they flush out toxins. Get plenty of water and herbal teas. Avoid caffeine and alcohol as they dehydrate. Also, it's important to consume enough electrolytes, especially for those who exercise often. You can get electrolytes from coconut water or sports drinks.

4. Avoid foods that can cause intolerance and allergic reactions

Certain foods can cause inflammation, leading to issues such as gas, bloating or diarrhea. Avoid certain foods if you have a food intolerance. These foods are common in fast-food establishments. All foods high in fat and salt like pizza, fries, or burgers, are high in sugar and salt. They also have chemicals that may cause inflammation.

5. Omega-3 Supplement

Omega-3 fatty oils are vital for overall health. They are particularly beneficial to people on high-dose dopamine. Supplement with a high-quality omega-3 supplement. Omega-3 rich foods include flaxseeds (chia seeds), salmon, walnuts, and chia seed. Supplements with fish oil and supplements of algae are other good sources.

6. Probiotics

Probiotics can help support gut health, while also allowing you to dopamine fast. The gut contains trillions, with some bacteria being beneficial and others not. Probiotics aid in maintaining a healthy amount of bacteria in your gut. They can also reduce inflammation and improve digestion. A probiotic should contain several strains of bacteria.

7. Avoid foods that contain high levels of lectin

Lectins are proteins that can be found in many foods. They can lead to digestive problems and inflammation. When dopamine fasting, avoid foods that contain lectins. These foods include grains, legumes and nightshade vegetable. Instead, try to eat nutrient rich fruits and veggies.

8. More Fermented Foods

Fermented foods have high amounts of probiotics that can aid in gut health. They also contain the essential enzymes for digestion. When you're dopamine fasting, try to include fermented food in your diet. Sauerkraut (kimchi), yogurt, and Kefir are good choices.

9. Increase your intake of healthy oils

Essential for your overall health, healthy fats play an important role. They improve brain function, support the immune systems, reduce inflammation and aid in weight loss. When fasting, increase your intake for healthy fats with foods such as nuts, olive oil, avocado, and seeds. You can also consume smoothies with healthy fats.

10. Avoid eating too late at night

It can cause sleep disruption and disrupt your dopamine fasting efforts. Avoid eating after 8pm. For a quick snack, eat a small amount of yogurt or fruit. To help digestion, take the time to thoroughly chew every food. You should make it a habit to eat slow and mindfully even when you're not fasting.

11. Exercise Regularly

Exercise is an excellent way to improve overall health. For people on fast dopamine, it's also very beneficial. Regular exercise can reduce inflammation and improve mood. It can also boost energy levels. You should aim to get at least 30 mins of exercise every day. It is also a great way to break up the monotony that comes with dieting. Diverse types of exercise are possible to keep things exciting.

12. Practice Mindfulness

Mindfulness is a meditation technique that can improve mental well being. It can also be beneficial to fasting individuals. Mindfulness can reduce anxiety, stress, and depression. It can also help with concentration and focus. For mindfulness, you need to find a calm place to sit or lie down. Keep your eyes closed and pay attention to your breathing. Take a moment to notice the thoughts and feelings that come to mind, but don't judge. Practice for 10-15 minutes per day.

Dopamine Fasting - The Benefits

Although it may seem like a new trend dopamine fasting is not a good idea for your overall health, there are some indications that it could be. Here are some of these benefits.

1. Focus and mental clarity are improved

Focus and mental clarity are two of the key benefits. Dopamine fasting prohibits the consumption of processed foods and sugary drinks. The body will function better if it's not being bombarded by processed food. When only healthy, nutritious foods are consumed, the mind is able to concentrate better and think clearly.

2. Low Inflammation

Chronic inflammation is linked with several health problems such as arthritis, cancer, heart disease and cancer. To improve your overall health, you must reduce inflammation. The elimination of processed foods and the inclusion of healthy fats can help reduce inflammation. You can get even more anti-inflammatory benefits from dopamine fasting if you add supplements such as fish oil and turmeric.

3. Weight Loss

This is an excellent way to lose fat. Weight loss will be inevitable when you focus on eating nutritious, high-quality foods. Dopamine fasting works well and is a lasting way to lose weight. This way of eating is not a temporary diet. It's a healthy and long-lasting way to eat.

4. Improved mood

Your mood can be negatively affected by processed foods. If you focus on eating nutritious, healthy foods, your mood is sure to improve. The body will no more be in a state that is toxic and it will be able work at its best. You'll notice an increase in energy and a decrease in mood swings.

5. Improved Digestion

Processed foods can have a negative impact on your digestive system. Eating healthy, fibrous foods will help improve digestion. Your dopamine fasting schedule will help you achieve optimal digestion. Regular exercise is an excellent way to get it done. You will also experience better digestion if you lose weight.

6. Energy consumption has increased

Consuming processed foods is high in sugar and caffeine which can lead to a decrease in energy levels. Energy levels will improve if you avoid processed foods and focus more on eating nutritious, healthy foods. You'll have more energy all day and be less likely to succumb to a mid-afternoon slump. Many people also report more energy when they do not take dopamine for a while.

7. Better Skin

Your skin is the largest organ on your body. Therefore, it is vital that you take care of it. Processed foods can damage skin health by causing dryness, wrinkles, and other problems. Healthy, nutrient-rich foods can help your skin become less oily. This will reduce the appearance of wrinkles and acne.

8. Lower risk of developing a disease

Consuming processed food increases your chance of developing chronic illnesses such as heart disease and cancer. Both excessive inflammation and the intake of unhealthy sugar are responsible. The anti-inflammatory effects of dopamine and the emphasis on healthy, nutrient-rich food can reduce the chance of these diseases.

9. Better Sleep

Processed foods can impact sleep quality and quantity. Inadequate sleep patterns can cause weight gain, increased disease risk, and other health problems. Healthy foods, such as those found in a fasting dopamine diet, can help promote healthy sleeping habits. You will notice a greater ease in falling asleep, and you'll sleep through the night with no wakeups.

10. Increased life span

Studies have shown that eating a healthy diet can help increase your lifespan. Healthy eating habits are essential to living a long, healthy life. This can be achieved by doing a dopamine fast. The benefits include better mental clarity, decreased inflammation, weight loss (weight loss), improved mood, and better digestion. It's worth it not only for addictive behavior, but also to lead a healthier and happier lifestyle.

Fasting Diets for Dopamine

While dopamine fasting is possible, there are many diets you can follow. Here are some of our most popular:

1. Paleo Diet

Paleo means that people are best suited to eat Paleolithic foods. It excludes processed foods, dairy and grains. Paleo emphasizes a healthy diet rich in nutrients, such as fruits, vegetables meat, poultry and seafood. You can modify the Paleo diet by avoiding starchy vegetables or consuming more healthy oils.

2. Mediterranean Diet

The Mediterranean diet was derived from the traditional Mediterranean diet. It is high on fruits, vegetables whole grains, legumes and fish. It is low on meat and processed foods. The Mediterranean diet is a great option for dopamine-free fasting. This is because it is nutrient dense and allows for flexibility in your food choices. Even if you don't eat meat or dairy, the Mediterranean diet can still be beneficial while you fast from dopamine.

3. Vegetarian Diet

A vegetarian diet is one that eliminates all animal products. This includes meat, poultry (seafood), eggs and seafood. There are many kinds of vegetarian diets. But most emphasize eating a variety fruits, vegetables, whole grain, and legumes. Dopamine fasting can be made easier by following a vegetarian diet. If you eat a vegetarian diet while on dopamine fast, you may feel more energetic and have better digestion.

4. Vegan Diet

Vegans are vegetarians who eat only plants and eliminate all animal products (meat, poultry, eggs, seafood, milk, etc.). It may be difficult for vegans to stick to a healthy lifestyle while fasting on dopamine. There aren't many options. With some creativity, you can maintain a healthy vegan lifestyle while still following dopamine fasting. Consider focusing your attention on nutrient rich foods like sweet potatoes, sweet potato, quinoa, and even chia seed.

5. Ketogenic Diet

The ketogenic is a high-fat and low-carbohydrate diet which helps induce ketosis. In ketosis, the body uses fat as energy instead of carbs. Because it is extremely restrictive, the ketogenic diet can be used to dopamine fasting. It is not easy to follow and may not be suitable for everyone.

6. Low-Carbohydrate Diet

A low-carbohydrate or carbohydrate diet refers to a diet that restricts how many carbohydrates you eat. Low-carbohydrate eating habits are popular for weight loss, and they are also effective for dopamine fasting. There are many low carbohydrate diets. But most emphasize eating healthy meats, vegetables and fruits.

7. Macronutrient Diet

A macronutrient-based diet considers the proportion of macronutrients consumed, such as carbohydrates (proteins, fats), and carbohydrates (carbohydrates). While a macronutrient fast can be maintained, it is important to ensure that your majority of calories come from healthy sources, such as fruits, vegetables and whole grains. Avoid fast food and candy.

8. Intermittent Fasting

Intermittent eating is a way to eat in a set time and then fast the rest of your day. Intermittent fasting may be used while on a dopamine-free fast. However, ensure you are getting the correct nutrients during your meal window. Your feeding window should be filled with nutrient-rich foods, such as fruits, vegetables and whole grains.

9. Juice Fast

A juice fast is when all food is juice. You can do a juice fast while fasting if your juice recipes include lots of healthy fruits and veggies. It is a great way of detoxifying your body and getting a variety nutrition. If you have an eating disorder, you should not follow this diet.

10. Bone Broth Fast

A bone-broth fast is one where bone broth is the only food consumed. Bone broth can be a healthy alternative to fasting because it is rich in nutrients and protein. When you dopamine fast, make sure to include plenty of vegetables. For athletes with ketogenic diets, bone broth fasts are often used to increase ketone and improve athletic performance.

Dopamine Fasting: A Fad or Real?

Dopamine fasting, which is a relatively new trend in the world of dopamine fasting, is still not well-known. But, evidence is mounting that it can be a very effective way to lose fat and improve your overall health. There are many ways to eat healthy, so it is flexible and can be followed on a variety of diets. It's not a fad since it has been around for awhile, is still popular, and works. This way of eating healthy will become more mainstream after further research on dopamine fasting.

Here are some key takeaways

Here's an overview of the contents of this chapter:

* Dopamine fasting, a diet and fasting strategy that focuses only on reducing the intake of dopamine inducing foods, is an approach to fasting.

There are many types and styles of dopaminefasting diets. However, most emphasize the importance of eating healthy foods like whole grains, fruits, and vegetables.

* Dopamine fasting can be adjusted by eating nutrients-rich foods such as fruits, vegetables and whole grains. Avoid unhealthy food like fast food and candy.

* Dopamine fasting is good for weight loss and improved mental clarity.

There are still questions as to whether dopamine-fasting is safe, but increasing evidence suggests that it can help you lose weight and improve your health.

* There are many diets that can be followed while fasting on dopamine, making it versatile and flexible in terms of healthy eating.

* Dopamine Fasting isn't a fad, but a growing trend. Further research is necessary to fully understand the effects dopamine fasting has on your body.

* Dopamine fasting may be done while you follow other types of diets so long as the majority of your calories are from healthy foods.

* Intermittent fasting can be done along with juice fasting and bone-broth fasting.

There are so many dopamine fasting options, it can be difficult for someone to choose the right one. Find the diet that best suits you and that you are able to maintain. If you don't know where to start, one of the dopaminefasting diets is a good place to start. Be sure to consult your doctor before trying any new diet.

5

Dopamine Detoxification - The Benefits

Now that you are familiar with the dopamine fasting and diet techniques, you might wonder if there is any real benefit to doing a dopamine detox. Depriving yourself from impulsive behaviours and denying yourself instant gratification can be hard work. It does. These benefits go beyond the mere ability to stop engaging mindless behavior (such as binge-watching television shows or scrolling on social networks), which is what most people are trying to achieve through dopamine detox.

You can't expect dopamine detox to solve all of your problems. Either way, you can't prevent every issue, person, event, or situation. This would hinder the normal release and cause a whole new set of problems. Therefore, it is best to work in small increments to get the benefits. Do not expect a quick fix to bring about long-term success. If we want to eliminate all distractions from our goals, we need to put in the effort to stop them. This is the topic we'll be discussing.

Freedom from Distractions

Our daily lives are filled with distractions, which we seem to gain much joy from. We can only see the lies in this false happiness when we distance ourselves from it. We begin to realize that dopamine only amplifies our enjoyment of certain activities. It is not the molecule with more because it doesn't have to. Dopamine encourages us all to seek repetition by engaging in activities that we find satisfying.

These distractions are harmful to your professional and personal development. Dopamine does not give us happiness if our brain doesn't produce as much dopamine. It provides us only with pleasure as a motivator, and not if we were seeking instant gratification. This is a great way to free yourself from distractions and allow you to pursue other valuable values that will benefit your mind and life.

This culture of distraction is something many people are involved in. It can be difficult to break free from. As you'll soon discover, the dopamine detox provides many other tools that you can use in your quest for freedom.

Teaches Discipline, and Freedom

While it may seem that independence and discipline are opposites, they can also be closely connected. In fact, the more independent someone is, the more they can have. Dopamine detox makes it easier to remove yourself from anything that could affect our willpower. When we dopamine detox, our self-control increases again, especially if mindfulness activities are included.

The solution to instant gratification lies in delaying it. This is something we can only do if our minds aren't flooded with high doses of dopamine. This will help us to understand that we can become more disciplined if we don't give in. This inner strength, however, is not something we were born with. Nor can we keep it without working hard to improve it. As with muscles, willpower gains strength through training. It is necessary to detoxify the dopamine first before we can train it.

Once that is done, we can choose how to become stronger. The way we choose to be stronger will depend on what our strengths, preferences, and other influences are revealed. Dopamine addicts can have difficulty with even small acts of self-discipline. The inability to resist instant gratification can cause willpower depletion. We will discuss this in the following chapters. Our freedom will increase if you can surpass this.

Comfort Zone expansion

Comfort zones revolve around what is familiar, and therefore safe. For example, it is much more safe to return to addictive dopamine-based behaviors than to pursue new experiences. However, continuing to engage in this addictive behavior will narrow our thinking and lead us to remain within our comfort zone. Despite the fact that we suffer the emotional and physical consequences from this narrow thought process we often are unable to admit that the reason we cannot get out is because of our addiction. We choose the safer way. We seek the same pleasures and dopamine shots to mask our feelings.

Dopamine detox can help us have new experiences and break our dependence on comfort. As a result, our comfort zone naturally expands and we feel more confident. You soon realize that many new things are only a few steps from your comfort zone. Even though it sounds scary, the best things in your life are not within your comfort zone.

It's often amazing what we can do beyond our comfort zones. They can teach us new lessons and allow us to grow. They help us realize that we should not let our goals or responsibilities slip by and be content.

Focus increases

We can focus better when we get away from our dopamine stimuli. We are able to concentrate on more tasks, and can approach them with greater intelligence. For example, most people are more productive in the first part of the day. However, their focus decreases over the course of the day. This is due to decision fatigue. Poor decisions are often made in this second half of the work day. It can lead to serious addiction and poor decision making. Because our brains are so overworked that we need a constant dopamine boost, it becomes a habit.

Our brains can go without dopamine when we detox. The more successful we are at detox, then the more we demonstrate that we can function without receiving any kind of gratification. This helps to eliminate all distractions, temptations, and makes it easier to stay focused. So, we have enough time for the more complicated tasks in our day.

It doesn't mean that our brains have to work too hard. This will allow us to make better decisions and reduce the risk of making mistakes. Now, we can focus on daily tasks, relationships and health, as well as the environment. It's far better than any stimulant, and it promises to ease the stress of a busy life.

Motivation

Even though our brains are highly developed and capable of managing many different processes at once dopamine forces us into irrational behavior. Dopamine causes us to indulge in dangerous vices that overpower our intrinsic self-motivational tools. While it might seem like we get our inspiration from the activities we enjoy, this is not a true motivation. To overcome this, our minds must be free from dopamine to allow us to see the potential and not feel motivated.

When our focus is improved, we find that we are more productive during the day. Contrary to dopamine, that is a pleasure that doesn't come with context, fulfilling responsibilities brings you real and lasting satisfaction. This makes it possible to take on more work at a professional level, and gain new skills that will help us improve our financial security.

Additionally, our dopamine-free brain encourages us set new goals in personal life. Our brains are free from dopamine, so we can set goals and work towards them without any distractions. We also have the ability to become more motivated to be a better person. While we all know that life is not easy and there are many things we should be concerned about, we can overcome these fears with true motivation.

Relaxes your Mind

Because we can do more work in a short time, there is more time to contemplate. It is rare that we are able to take the time to reflect, contemplate our choices, or wonder beyond our current circumstances. We don't do this often anymore. We live busy, so whenever we have some spare time, we reach out for the tool to give us the dopamine boost and distract from these questions.

All the stimuli our brains receive from different sources makes it hard for us to relax enough to consider anything meaningful. It's too busy scrolling through social media and all the other media. While we all know that some content can be negative, we still love the dopamine-releasing effects. While we all know that these dopamine shot should not be used as crutches we cannot help but feel the need to use them.

It is possible to think about everything you want when we remove the tools that provide this release. It's possible to do this while sitting in line or waiting in the park during lunch - all the time that we normally spend searching for the dopamine inducing pleasure of your choice. Dopamine detox lets us reclaim this time to ourselves. We can now focus on our present and future lives, what we can contribute to the world, and so much more.

Helps to Set Goals

We have been taught to see only short-term goals because of our fast-paced culture. This is what makes us addicted to instant gratification. With mindfulness exercises and other dopamine detox strategies, we can overcome this mindset. At the same time, mindfulness exercises and other dopamine detox techniques can help us focus and be more productive. We also discover that patience is a highly valued virtue that offers many benefits.

A great way to boost productivity is to set short-term goals. These short-term goals make us more confident in setting long-term ones. These give us more satisfaction and fulfillment, in whatever area of life. Our ability to accomplish great things is enhanced when we don't have anxiety or distractions.

But, these benefits can only come from healthy dopamine detox. A lack of dopamine detox could lead to the elimination of all sources of pleasure, which can again cause unhappiness and productivity. It is much easier to find ways to have short-term happiness while living a healthier lifestyle. This will increase our chances of improving our long-term lives.

Creativity rises

Focusing on the source for dopamine release (such social media) is the only way to get it. Since we know we will only get the shot when we act in certain ways, we are unable to engage in creative thinking. For us to eat, we don't necessarily need vision. It isn't true. Our greatest strength may be our imagination.

In addition to contemplating our choices and goals, we can also be alone and dream, imagine, think, and eventually achieve greatness in life. This is possible if we allow our brain to become independent of the dopamine release source. Dopamine detox allows us to regain this ability even though it may seem impossible.

Sometimes, people are unaware of their creative potential until they tap into that creativity by trying a new approach to a difficult assignment or creating a new hobby. Our solitude can be re-evaluated when we have no dopamine. Instead of seeing them negatively, try to use them to create new ideas and perspectives.

Improves our mood

Spirituality will tell you that it's not surprising that we attract positive energy when our vibrations are higher. Although it is linked to health benefits this vibration can also have other effects - at the very least in the dopamine loop. Even if there are no mental health issues, dopamine levels that fluctuate between highs or lows can have a profound impact on our mood.

The tool that triggers our brain to release dopamine immediately is often used to improve our mood. Dopamine levels in the body drop immediately after instant gratification. This vicious cycle is repeated as we continue to search for the source of the empty release.

Dopamine detox can help you get rid of these symptoms. While this can be difficult, it will allow you to stabilize your mood over the long-term and help you make positive life changes. There is no better way than to improve our mood, but to see our goals achieved after many productive hours - not the days wasted on pleasure-seeking activities but for the detox.

Tames Unhealthy Desires

Dopamine is just another chemical that drives us back to it no matter how many times. It makes dopamine-induced pleasure very difficult to avoid. In the end, it becomes so overwhelming that we cannot avoid it at all. The release will erase any benefit we may have gained, and leave behind a vast void.

Dopamine detox helps to eliminate the causes of these desires and allows us to let go of the things that control our daily life. Because we are now forced to re-evaluate how our emotions affect our emotional regulation, it also improves our emotional regulation.

When we get rid of toxic sources, our emotional life is more controlled, peaceful, as well as pain-free.

This detox increases our resistance to temptation from the same guilty pleasures which hooked us up on the dopamine system. When we find ourselves in a dopamine-inducing temptation to grab another drug, we will be able rethink our decision and stop reaching for it. It is important to choose positive actions to lead a fulfilling and happy life. These can be more difficult than usual, but the rewards for making them are much greater.

Satisfaction increases

If we aren't able to have a fulfilling, happy life, it is difficult to expect to be fulfilled. Our comfort zone is often a key factor in our life satisfaction. One aspect of dopamine withdrawal is how we can achieve the best level of happiness with our choices and our lives in general. Dopamine detox removes our worries and other stress factors. This allows us to experience a state where everything is more positive.

One of the benefits of a dopamine free mind is being able to look back on past actions and see their consequences. If we look back at a negative event, we can learn from it and not focus on the pain. As it is not possible to eliminate all of the enjoyable experiences from our lives it is also impossible to remove the negative ones.

The only way to win in this world, where there are so many temptations to distract and cause grief in different ways, is to dopamine detox. It allows us to control our behavior and avoid any situations that might be out of our hands. It allows one to achieve long-term, ultimate satisfaction.

Promotes Healthier Relationships

Every day we learn new ways of being socially acceptable. But not all of them can be good for us. The dopamine that we get from accepting these behaviors can give rise to a false sense or happiness. It also leads to unhealthy relationships and dopamine releases. While it is difficult at first to receive dopamine release or a response, we soon discover the mistake we made in relationships that matter.

Whatever addictive behavior you're struggling with, social media can help. If you can let it go for a while, it will be easier to see its true effects and will lead to a healthier relationship. Breaking the cycle of compulsive behaviors can help you to desire to change far more than just our digital relationships or social media. This is a good starting point in learning about addiction.

But, in order to live a happier life, we need to establish healthier relationships with our environment. Dopamine detox can help. You know what it means to pay more attention? It makes you better at communicating your emotions. This is not a coincidence. This is not a coincidence. When compulsive behavior isn't distracting, we can concentrate on our relationships. If people notice how much we care about them and don't lose ourselves in our world, then they will reciprocate. This will lead to deeper relationships.

Physical and Mental Health Improvements

It is a sign of our ability to deal with potentially problematic behavior if we go the extra mile to achieve these goals. All of our bad behavior patterns are caused by a dopamine addiction. Dopamine addictions can cause a poor mental state, which can lead to negative behavior patterns. It is worth reducing high doses. Our state of mind can often impact the health of our body - and we may be able now to overcome potential health issues.

It is possible to be more present without any distractions, such as a screen or substance. It may seem frightening to some at first. Everyone can overcome any obstacle with determination and motivation.

Our spiritual energy (vibe, or vibration), will rise as we improve both our mental and our physical health. The many distractions can cause our vibrational energy to become out-of-balance. This can lead, as we've already seen, to many of these issues. If we can get out of this constant dopamine loop we can increase our vibe and attract positive and productive energy into your life. We begin to notice the positive changes healthier habits bring. It is all because our brains aren't being bombarded anymore with this addictive chemical.

Here are some key takeaways

Dopamine detoxes are beneficial when done in a healthy way.

* Long-term-benefits may also be possible, but this takes a lot more time and effort. These benefits can only be obtained if we have the patience.

* Dopamine detox's most significant advantage is its paradox of freedom providing

discipline. The more you discipline yourself, the more freedom you have to do whatever you like in life.

* We have the freedom to be free from an unhealthy culture that is full of distractions.

* Lack of dopamine means that we should not give in to our urges. Sometimes, it's necessary to learn how to control our passions in order not let them devour us.

* Avoiding triggers will allow our mind to be focused on the present activities, and our physical and spiritual well-being.

* Now that we don't get bombarded constantly with dopamine release, we can pay attention to our vibe and energy more.

* By removing distractions from our lives, we can begin to think about different aspects of our lives and make the necessary changes.

* Having a better sense of focus helps us to be more focused and motivated to succeed in

life. We learn how to set long-term and short-term goals.

* We have more time for creativity and can even explore new career options or hobbies.

* Unable to enjoy certain pleasures will force us to try new ones. This often forces us to step outside of our comfort zone but also allows us the opportunity to learn new things.

* If we are unable to satisfy our immediate needs, we can discover more joys in life. This includes the importance of having better relationships with our surrounding environment.

* The brain still produces dopamine, but in smaller amounts. This means that detoxing from it takes a special approach. Next chapter will explain how to fully detoxify your brain's production of dopamine.

6

Methods and Strategies to Completely Detoxify Your Brain's Dopamine Productivity

In the previous chapters we have explored the notion of addiction and discussed dopamine fasting, which is a viable option to break the harmful cycle. But you might still be unsure. How can we effectively let go the things that give rise to dopamine and bring us instant happiness? It will not be easy. Unfortunately, the digital world has been designed to exploit dopamine systems. With the right strategies and dedication, you can change those unhealthy habits.

Modern technology can reinforce many of the most prevalent addictions. The modern world is fast-paced and stressful, so we need to find cheap and readily available dopamine. Before we know, our society has become dependent on these temporary escapism and happiness methods.

A dopamine detox can help with your addictions. This is when you are able to change your behavior and adopt healthier, more fulfilling habits. This will replace the addictive pleasures you feel with the pleasure you get from new behaviors, activities, and experiences. The added benefit is that your new ventures can give you long-lasting contentment rather than the quick fix dopamine hit you received in the past. This chapter provides information on dopamine detox as well as tips and rules to help you succeed. It provides you with many strategies and helpful tips that will help you to break bad habits.

It works

Remember that there is no single right way to "dopamine detox". There are many ways to approach it, depending on personal factors. Each person is different. We all react differently to the same situations. You may find that what works for one person doesn't work for you. This means that you may have to spend a lot of time thinking about what works for you and trying different techniques. You don't have to worry, because we're here for you. However, before we go into detail about the strategies available to you, we must first explain their operation.

You're trying to get rid off repetitive behaviors. Therefore, you can refer to them as "loops." A behavior loop is an action where a person experiences a trigger, responds with a particular action, and then triggers another response. The response that is favorable, such as a positive dopamine hit is reinforced in your case. There are generally two types, engagement loops or escape loops.

Escape Loops are for unwanted behavior

An escape loop can be defined as any activity or situation in your daily life that offers low-value contentment and pleasure. These escape loops are marked by the quick, cheap, and easy dopamine hit they provide. This is a typical escape loop.

You may experience negative emotions, such as sadness or boredom, and even anxiety. It can make you feel unhappy or unfulfilled. It can be accompanied with low-level stress levels and increases in cortisol. The uncomfortable feelings are what you want to change. There are two options. One is to identify the root of the problem, fix it (which can often be more time-consuming and costly), or find a more cost-effective, faster and more convenient way to get dopamine flowing again.

When you engage in this "escape" or behavior, it makes you feel joyful. Once you feel triggered, you'll decide to do this again. Your brain tricks yourself into believing that it is in control. For that moment of extreme pleasure, however, you will eventually rely on your brain. You are in a feedback loop that is dependent before you know.

Escape loops can be used to avoid the root cause of the problem. This escape plan lets you skip all the work of fixing the problem to feel better. Even if the pleasure is short-lived and you are aware of its dangers, it can still be appealing to many people. This behavior is not only very bad for your mental, emotional, and physical health, but also causes you to feel horrible after experiencing that brief pleasure. It is a destructive loop that leads to your own destruction.

Instead of finding a hobby, many people reach for their phones whenever they feel bored. People who dislike their jobs may choose to drown their sorrows by looking for new opportunities. People who feel lonely may turn to porn in order to fill the temporary void. While each person may have a different escape loop, all of them are destructive.

What is the solution?

Engaging in Unwanted Behaviors

As you can see an engagement loop works in the same way as an escape loop. Instead of allowing yourself the quick dopamine fix, force yourself to wait so you can create richer, more meaningful experiences in your life. If you don't make this conscious decision, you risk falling into the traps of the digital age.

As we said, engaging in a loop is more challenging and costly than not engaging, especially if there is an addiction. These engaging behaviors are those that everyone wants to do but isn't able to. After a long work day, it's natural to want to get out of your comfort zone and go running, to the gym or to meet people.

Sometimes, you feel like this is not a big deal. You might scroll through your Instagram feed for a few minutes prior to your friends arrive or you may have just one beer on a night out. It doesn't always work like that. It doesn't matter how small your actions are, they serve as foundations for the life that you build for yourself. A good life will be built by smart and conscious choices and positive actions. Harmful people, especially those you are struggling with, will hinder the future you want to create.

We've already examined the typical escape circuit. How does an engagement ring look?

You feel sad, anxious, bored, or lonely. This feeling is unfulfilling and can lead to low-level stress. You feel depressed and unfulfilled. This means you are willing to tackle the difficult task of fixing it. It will make you feel better about yourself and the decisions you make. It is a wonderful feeling to achieve something, and it's a joy to be able to make positive decisions.

Engagement loops are difficult to sustain. Engagement loops require constant effort, dedication and motivation as well hard work. Once established, they offer a deep feeling of fulfillment, meaning, and satisfaction. They allow you to make lasting life changes and redefine your purpose. Each person has a unique engagement loop. It is important to choose a method or activity that will sustain your loop for the long term. An example of an engagement loop is disconnecting with the digital world, connecting to others in person and reading, as well as eating a healthy diet and engaging in physical activities.

Establishing an Engagement Chain

Introspection is a key part of creating an engagement circle. First, determine why you feel this way. Then identify your favorite escapes and behaviors. Do you have a problem? This behavior could be linked to past traumas, psychological issues or other factors. Also, do you know why this habit developed? Look at where you're hiding from responsibility and consider how your future self will be affected. What can you do to reach your goals?

Look at the problems you often face in life. Reflect on your failures and mistakes in the past to help you become a better person. Think about how these past experiences may have influenced your approach to obstacles. Face the root causes and be open to them. These are the things you will need to confront throughout your journey. You will find solutions that you don't want to address and so you need an escape plan.

If you have multiple escape options, try to focus on one. It doesn't mean that you have to keep to one loop for each unwanted behavior. One positive engagement may be your best option. It will give you large amounts of dopamine and last a long time. The more complicated your relationships are, the easier it will be for you to maintain these lifestyle changes.

Visualize Your Future

Imagine yourself 5-10 years from now. Take as much time and as many as you want. Take down all the thoughts that come to your mind. Visualize every detail. Think about your home, the way it's decorated, your appearance, what you wear, and how your car looks. If you have a family, consider your relationship with them as well as how you interact. Consider the amount of time you have with them, and what activities you do together. What is your job? Which office do you work in? What's the look of your office? What's your average workday like? What about your eating habits? Are you vegan or vegetarian? Are you eating a healthy, balanced diet? You may go to the gym but you aren't losing weight. What are your favorite activities? Are you interested in taking care of them professionally? Are you a pet-owner? Do you travel regularly?

You now know how you want your future. Now think about your current life. What steps can you take to get there? Can your escape loop help get you there? If it doesn't, what will stop you? What does the ideal engagement loop look like? What activities and what kind of lifestyle can help you achieve this? This isn't meant to make anyone feel overwhelmed. These changes are not necessary overnight. That would be impossible. These are the things that matter. You can always turn to your ideal, future self for motivation whenever you feel the need to move ahead.

Detoxing

There are no strict rules to dopamine detox. The length of your detox will determine how effective it is. You should do a deep detox, which will allow you to break all bad habits. But many prefer to detoxify their brains first for a set amount of time. Remember that these 24-hour and 30-day detoxes target multiple areas of your life instead of just one. Temporary lifestyle changes may not be enough to keep you from falling for the same traps and causing the same problems down the road.

The 24-hour detox can be very difficult and therefore is not sustainable. If you don't do a follow up detox plan, the 24-hour detox will have very limited impact. Many people struggle to integrate the 30-day detox into their lifestyle.